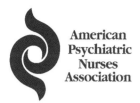
American
Psychiatric
Nurses
Association

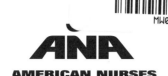
AMERICAN NURSES
ASSOCIATION

ISPN

MW01046633

PSYCHIATRIC-MENTAL HEALTH
NURSING:
SCOPE AND STANDARDS
OF PRACTICE

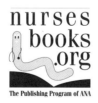
nurses
books
.org
The Publishing Program of ANA

AMERICAN PSYCHIATRIC NURSES ASSOCIATION
INTERNATIONAL SOCIETY OF PSYCHIATRIC-MENTAL HEALTH NURSES

AMERICAN NURSES ASSOCIATION
SILVER SPRING, MARYLAND
2007

Library of Congress Cataloging-in-Publication data

Psychiatric-mental health nursing : scope and standards of practice / American Psychiatric Nurses Association, International Society of Psychiatric-Mental Health Nurses.
    p. ; cm.
    Includes bibliographical references and index.
    ISBN-13: 978-1-55810-250-7 (pbk. : alk. paper)
    ISBN-10: 1-55810-250-7 (pbk. : alk. paper)
    1. Psychiatric nursing.   2. Psychiatric nursing—Standards.   I. American Psychiatric Nurses Association.   II. International Society of Psychiatric-Mental Health Nurses. III. American Nurses Association.
    [DNLM: 1. Psychiatric Nursing—methods—United States.   2. Psychiatric Nursing standards—United States.   3. Ethics, Nursing—United States.
WY 160 P974 2007]

RC440.P7599 2007
    616.89'0231—dc22   2007009743

The American Nurses Association (ANA) is a national professional association. This ANA publication— *Psychiatric-Mental Health Nursing: Scope and Standards of Practice*—reflects the thinking of the nursing profession on various issues and should be reviewed in conjunction with state board of nursing policies and practices. State law, rules, and regulations govern the practice of nursing, while *Psychiatric-Mental Health Nursing: Scope and Standards of Practice* guides nurses in the application of their professional skills and responsibilities.

Published by Nursesbooks.org
The Publishing Program of ANA

American Nurses Association
8515 Georgia Avenue, Suite 400
Silver Spring, MD 20910-3492
1-800-274-4ANA
http://www.nursesbooks.org/

ANA is the only full-service professional organization representing the nation's 2.9 million Registered Nurses through its 54 constituent member associations. ANA advances the nursing profession by fostering high standards of nursing practice, promoting the economic and general welfare of nurses in the workplace, projecting a positive and realistic view of nursing, and lobbying the Congress and regulatory agencies on healthcare issues affecting nurses and the public.

Design: Scott Bell, Arlington, VA; Freedom by Design, Alexandria, VA; Stacy Maguire, Sterling, VA ~ *Composition*: House of Equations, Inc., Arden, NC ~ *Editing and Indexing*: Steven A. Jent, Denton, TX ~ *Proofreading:* Lisa Munsat Anthony, Chapel Hill, NC ~ *Printing*: McArdle Printing, Upper Marlboro, MD

First printing May 2007.

ISBN-13: 978-1-55810-250-7   ISBN-10: 1-55810-250-7   SAN: 851-3481
07SSPMH   5M   05/07

ACKNOWLEDGMENTS

Work Group Members

Carole Farley-Toombs, MS, RN, CNAA, BC, Co-Chair
Peggy Dulaney, MSN, RN, BC, Co-Chair
Kathleen Delaney, PhD, APRN, BC
Judi Haber, PhD, APRN, BC, FAAN
Lynette Jack, PhD, RN
Ellen Mahoney, DNSc, APRN, BC
Colleen Parsons, RN, C
Beth Phoenix, PhD, RN
Larry Plant, MS, PMH-NP, APRN, BC
Peggy Plunkett, MSN, APRN, BC
Diane Snow, PhD, APRN, BC, CARN, PMHNP
Sandra Talley, PhD, APRN, BC, FAAN
Christine Tebaldi, MS, APRN, BC
Karen Ballard, MA, RN, Consultant

ANA Staff

Carol J. Bickford, PhD, RN, BC—Content editor
Yvonne Daley Humes, MSA—Project coordinator
Matthew Seiler, RN, Esq.—Legal counsel

Winifred Carson-Smith, JD—Consultant

The American Psychiatric Nurses Association (APNA) is a professional membership organization committed to the specialty practice of psychiatric mental health nursing, health and wellness promotion through identification of mental health issues, prevention of mental health problems, and the care and treatment of persons with psychiatric disorders. http://www.apna-psych.org

The International Society of Psychiatric-Mental Health Nurses (ISPN) exists to unite and strengthen the presence and the voice of specialty psychiatric-mental health nursing while influencing healthcare policy to promote equitable, evidence-based and effective treatment and care for individuals, families, and communities. http://www.ispn-psych.org

CONTENTS

Acknowledgments   iii

Preface   vii

Psychiatric-Mental Health Nursing: Scope of Practice   1
Introduction   1
History and Evolution of the Specialty   2
Origins of the Advanced Practice Psychiatric-Mental Health   3
     Nursing Role
Current Issues and Trends   5
     Prevalence of Mental Disorders Across the Lifespan   6
     Disparities among Diverse Populations   7
     Psychiatric-Mental Health Nursing Leadership in   8
          Transforming the Mental Health System
     Prevention   11
     The Evolving Role of National Data Systems to Improve Quality   11
     Evidence-Based Practice and Lifelong Learning   12
     Safety for Patients and for PMH Nurses   13
Definition of Psychiatric-Mental Health Nursing   13
Phenomena of Concern for Psychiatric-Mental Health Nurses   15
Levels of Psychiatric-Mental Health Nursing Practice   16
     Psychiatric-Mental Health Registered Nurse (RN-PMH)   16
     Psychiatric-Mental Health Advanced Practice Registered   19
          Nurse (APRN-PMH)
     Psychotherapy   20
     Psychopharmacological Interventions   21
     Case Management   21
     Program Development and Management   21
     Consultation and Liaison   22
     Clinical Supervision   22
Ethical Issues in Psychiatric-Mental Health Nursing   23
Specialized Areas of Practice   23
     Psychiatric-Mental Health Nursing Clinical Practice Settings   23
     Crisis Intervention and Psychiatric Emergency Services   24
     Acute Inpatient Care   24
     Intermediate and Long-Term Care   24
     Partial Hospitalization and Intensive Outpatient Treatment   24
     Residential Services   25

Community-Based Care   25
Assertive Community Treatment (ACT)   25
Primary Care   25
Integrative Programs   26
Telehealth   26
Self-Employment   27
Forensic Mental Health   27
Disaster Mental Health   28

Standards of Practice   **29**
Standard 1. Assessment   29
Standard 2. Diagnosis   31
Standard 3. Outcomes Identification   32
Standard 4. Planning   33
Standard 5. Implementation   35
   Standard 5a. Coordination of Care   36
   Standard 5b. Health Teaching and Health Promotion 37
   Standard 5c. Milieu Therapy   39
   Standard 5d. Pharmacological, Biological, and Integrative   40
     Therapies
   Standard 5e. Prescriptive Authority and Treatment 41
   Standard 5f.   Psychotherapy   42
   Standard 5g. Consultation   43
Standard 6. Evaluation   44

Standards of Professional Performance   **45**
Standard 7. Quality of Practice   45
Standard 8. Education   47
Standard 9. Professional Practice Evaluation   48
Standard 10. Collegiality   49
Standard 11. Collaboration   50
Standard 12. Ethics   51
Standard 13. Research   52
Standard 14. Resource Utilization   53
Standard 15. Leadership   54

References   **57**

Glossary   **65**

Appendix A. *Scope and Standards of Psychiatric-*   **69**
Mental Health Nursing Practice **(2000)**

Index   **139**

PREFACE

The American Nursing Association's Congress on Nursing Practice and Economics is responsible for ensuring the relevance of published scope and standards and requires review of such documents every five years. In early 2004, the American Psychiatric Nurses Association and the International Society of Psychiatric-Mental Health Nurses appointed a joint task force to begin the review and revision of the *Scope and Standards of Psychiatric-Mental Health Nursing Practice* published in 2000 by the American Nurses Association (ANA, 2000).

A panel of psychiatric-mental health nursing experts and ANA policy leaders convened in August, 2005, to review initial drafts and make recommendations. The panel members held leadership positions as psychiatric-mental health nursing experts in various nursing organizations, including the American Psychiatric Nurses Association, the International Society of Psychiatric-Mental Health Nurses, the American Academy of Nursing, the Child and Adolescent (ACAPN) Division of the International Society of Psychiatric-Mental Health Nurses, the National Organization of Nurse Practitioner Faculty, and the International Nursing Society on Addictions. The panel members represented psychiatric-mental health nursing clinical administrators, staff nurses, and psychiatric advanced practice nurses working in acute psychiatric care settings.

In accordance with their recommendations, this document reflects the template language of the most recent publication of ANA nursing standards, *Nursing: Scope and Standards of Practice* (ANA, 2004). In addition, the introduction has been revised to highlight the leadership role of psychiatric-mental health nurses in the transformation of the mental health system as outlined in the President's New Freedom Commission Report of 2003 (New Freedom Commission, 2003). The prevalence of mental health issues and psychiatric disorders across the age span and the disparities in access to care and treatment among diverse groups attest the critical role that the specialty of psychiatric-mental health nursing must continue to play in meeting the goals for a healthy society. Safety issues for patients with psychiatric disorders and the nurses involved in their care are major priorities for this nursing specialty in an environment of fiscal constraints and disparities in reimbursement for mental health services.

Development of *Psychiatric-Mental Health Nursing: Scope and Standards of Practice* included a two-stage field review process: 1) review and feedback from the boards of the American Psychiatric Nurses Association and the International Society of Psychiatric-Mental Health Nursing and 2) posting of the draft for public comment at http://www.ISPN-psych.org with links from the ANA website, http://nursingworld.org, and the APNA website, http://www.apna.org. Notice of the public comment period was distributed to nursing specialty organizations, state boards of nursing, schools of nursing, faculty groups, and state nurses associations. All groups were encouraged to disseminate notice of the postings to all of their members and other stakeholders. Ninety-three people registered on the website during the posting period. Twenty-one comments and suggestions were received from individuals, faculty groups, and state nurses association psychiatric nursing groups. The feedback was carefully reviewed and integrated as appropriate.

Psychiatric-Mental Health Nursing: Scope of Practice

Psychiatric-mental health nursing is a specialized area of nursing practice committed to promoting mental health through the assessment, diagnosis, and treatment of human responses to mental health problems and psychiatric disorders. Psychiatric-mental health nursing, a core mental health profession, employs a purposeful use of self as its art and a wide range of nursing, psychosocial, and neurobiological theories and research evidence as its science.

Introduction

The nursing profession, by developing and articulating the scope and standards of professional nursing practice, defines its boundaries and informs society about the parameters of nursing practice. The scope and standards also guide the development of state-level nurse practice acts and the rules and regulations governing nursing practice.

Because each state develops its own regulatory language about nursing, the designated limits, functions, and titles for nurses, particularly at the advanced practice level, may differ significantly from state to state. Nurses must ensure that their practice remains within the boundaries defined by their state practice acts. Individual nurses are accountable for ensuring that they practice within the limits of their own competency, professional code of ethics, and professional practice standards.

Levels of nursing practice are differentiated according to the nurse's educational preparation. The nurse's role, position, job description, and work practice setting further define practice. The nurse's role may be focused on clinical practice, administration, education, or research.

This document addresses the role, scope of practice, and standards of practice specific to the specialty practice of psychiatric-mental health nursing. The scope statement defines psychiatric-mental health nursing and describes its evolution as a nursing specialty, its levels of practice based on educational preparation, current clinical practice activities and sites, and current trends and issues relevant to the practice of psychiatric-mental health nursing. The standards of psychiatric-mental health nursing practice are authoritative statements by which the psychiatric-mental health nursing specialty describes the responsibilities for which its practitioners are accountable.

History and Evolution of the Specialty

Psychiatric-mental health nursing as a specialty has its roots in nineteenth-century reform movements to reorganize mental asylums into hospitalized settings and to develop care and treatment for the mentally ill (Church, 1982). The first organized efforts to develop psychiatric nursing started at McLean Asylum in Massachusetts in 1882. Early nursing leaders such as Harriet Bailey, Euphemia Jane Taylor, and Lillian Wald supported the Mental Hygiene Movement and advocated for the acceptance of the emerging specialty of psychiatric nursing into the larger community of general nursing. The first nurse-organized training program for psychiatric nursing within a general nursing education program was established at Phipps Clinic at Johns Hopkins Hospital in 1913. This served as the prototype for other nursing education programs (Buckwalter & Church, 1979).

Under nursing leadership, psychiatric-mental health nursing evolved from the narrow focus of medical models and mind–body dichotomy towards a biopsychosocial approach to mental illness, including the concept of mind as expressed in behavior and adaptation to experience (Church, 1982). Psychiatric-mental health nursing leaders played a critical role in identifying and developing relevant specialized bodies of knowledge and in securing the didactic and clinical experiences necessary for students to achieve competence as mental health nurses.

The successful promotion of the integration of mental health concepts into general nursing educational programs facilitated a national public awareness of the relationship between mental and physical health in achieving patient outcomes. Through such efforts, psychiatric-mental health nursing practice moved far beyond the walls of state hospital institutions to meet the mental health needs of the community (Church, 1982). This more visible position became extremely important when the next wave of reform occurred in the 1940s with the passage of the National Mental Health Act and the development of nursing graduate programs in psychiatric-mental health nursing.

Many nurses entered graduate programs in psychiatric-mental health nursing once they became available beginning in 1954. However, registered nurses prepared at the undergraduate level continued to practice within the specialty of psychiatric-mental health nursing, primarily in hospital-based and psychiatric acute care settings. In recognition of this specialty nursing practice, the American Nurses Credentialing Center (ANCC) began to offer certification in psychiatric-mental health nursing at the undergraduate level in 1979. As the locus of care moved towards community-based programs, psychiatric-mental health nurses continued to develop their role to meet the needs of patients across the entire spectrum of care including continuing day treatment programs and group homes.

Origins of the Advanced Practice Psychiatric-Mental Health Nursing Role

Specialty nursing at the graduate level began to evolve in the late 1950s in response to the passage of the National Mental Health Act of 1946 and the creation of the National Institute of Mental Health in 1949. The National Mental Health Act of 1946 identified psychiatric nursing as one of four core disciplines for the provision of psychiatric care and treatment, along with psychiatry, psychology, and social work. Nurses played an active role in meeting the growing demand for psychiatric services that resulted from increasing awareness of post-war mental health issues (Bigbee & Amidi-Nouri, 2000). The incidence of "battle fatigue" led to the recognition of the need for more mental health professionals.

The first specialty degree in psychiatric-mental health nursing, a master's degree, was awarded at Rutgers University in 1954 under the leadership of Hildegard Peplau. In contrast to existing graduate nursing programs that focused on developing educators and consultants, graduate education in psychiatric-mental health nursing was designed to prepare nurse therapists to assess and diagnose mental health problems and psychiatric disorders, and provide individual, group, and family therapy. Psychiatric nurses pioneered the development of the advanced practice nursing role and led in establishing national specialty certification through the American Nurses Association.

The Community Mental Health Centers Act of 1963 facilitated the expansion of psychiatric Clinical Nurse Specialist (CNS) practice into outpatient and ambulatory care sites. These master's and doctorally pre-pared CNSs fulfilled a crucial role in helping deinstitutionalized mentally ill persons adapt to community life. Traineeships to fund graduate edu-cation provided through the National Institute of Mental Health played a significant role in expanding the psychiatric Clinical Nurse Specialist workforce. By the late 1960s they were providing individual, group, and family psychotherapy in a broad range of settings and obtaining third-party reimbursement. Psychiatric Clinical Nurse Specialists were also functioning as educators, researchers, and managers, and working in consultation-liaison positions or in the area of addictions. These roles continue today.

Another paradigm shift occurred as research renewed the emphasis on the neurobiologic basis of mental illness and addiction. As more efficacious psychotropic medications with fewer side effects were de-veloped, psychopharmacology assumed a more central role in psychi-atric treatment. The role of the psychiatric-mental health Clinical Nurse Specialist evolved to encompass the expanding biopsychosocial per-spective, and the competencies required for practice were kept congru-ent with emerging science. Many psychiatric graduate nursing programs added neurobiology, advanced health assessment, pharmacology, pathophysiology, and the diagnosis and medical management of psychiatric illness to their curricula. Similarly, preparation for prescrip-tive privileges became embedded in advanced practice psychiatric-mental health nursing graduate programs (Kaas & Markley, 1998).

Other trends in mental health and the larger healthcare system sparked other significant changes in advanced practice psychiatric nurs-ing. These trends included:

- A shift in National Institute of Mental Health (NIMH) funds from education to research, leading to a dramatic decline in enrollment in psychiatric nursing graduate programs (Taylor, 1999).

- An increased awareness of physical health problems in mentally ill persons living in community settings (Chafetz et al., 2005).

- The shift to primary care as a primary point of entry for compre-hensive health care, including psychiatric specialty care.

- The growth and public recognition of the nurse practitioner role in primary care settings.

In response to these challenges, psychiatric nursing graduate programs changed their curricula to include greater emphasis on comprehensive health assessment and referral and management of common physical health problems, and a continued focus on educational preparation to meet the state criteria and professional competencies for prescriptive authority. The tremendous expansion in the use of nurse practitioners in primary care settings had made *Nurse Practitioner* synonymous with *advanced practice nurse* for many in the general public and in some state practice acts. Although psychiatric-mental health nursing was not seeking a title change (Bjorklund, 2003), the specialty found itself drawn toward the use of the title Nurse Practitioner in response to market forces and state regulations (Wheeler & Haber, 2004; Delaney et al., 1999). The Psychiatric-Mental Health Nurse Practitioner role was clearly delineated by the publication of the *Psychiatric-Mental Health Nurse Practitioner Competencies* (National Panel, 2003), the product of a panel with representation from a broad base of nursing organizations sponsored by the National Organization of Nurse Practitioner Faculty.

Psychiatric-Mental Health Advanced Practice Nurses, whether they practice under the title of CNS or NP, share the same core competencies of clinical and professional practice. This is reflected in the core curriculum of graduate Psychiatric-Mental Health Nursing programs. Since there is little evidence of consistent differences in these roles nationwide, support has grown within the specialty for use of the term Advanced Practice Registered Nurse–Psychiatric-Mental Health (APRN-PMH) as the preferred title for advanced practice psychiatric nursing. ANA identifies Advanced Practice Registered Nurses (APRNs) as professional nurses who have successfully completed a graduate program of study in a nursing specialty that provides specialized knowledge and skills that form the foundation for expanded roles in health care.

Current Issues and Trends

Major changes in the healthcare delivery system, practice patterns of health professionals, and funding continue to have a profound effect on mental health care and psychiatric-mental health nursing practice. Nationally, healthcare delivery systems, educational institutions, policy makers, and health professionals have been challenged to create a vision for mental healthcare delivery that reduces health disparities and embeds quality, safety, evidence-based practice, inter-professional practice, and cultural competence as essential dimensions of consumer-focused twenty-first-century mental healthcare delivery and professional practice (New Freedom Commission on Mental Health, 2003; Daniels & Adams, 2004).

Prevalence of Mental Disorders Across the Lifespan

Because mental disorders are a major health problem in the United States and internationally, a challenge has been issued to all core health professions to identify, treat, and prevent mental illness. An estimated 22% of Americans aged 18 and older, about one in five adults, suffer from a diagnosable psychiatric disorder at any given time. Based on the 1998 U.S. Census residential population estimate, this figure translates to some 44.3 million people.

The World Health Organization (WHO, 2002) cites depression as the number one health problem worldwide. Approximately 15% of the population with a medical illness has co-occurring psychiatric illnesses. This co-morbidity predisposes them to a persistent course of chronic illness and increased utilization of mental health and other resources. Furthermore, four of the ten leading causes of disability in the United States and other developed countries are psychiatric disorders, namely major depression, bipolar disorder, schizophrenia, and anxiety disorders. WHO (2001) reports that psychiatric disorders account for 24% of all health-related disability, 12% of alcohol and drug use disorders, and 7% of Alzheimer's and dementias. Adding these categories together allows one to conclude that fully 43% of all health-related disability is directly due to psychiatric disorders.

The overall prevalence of psychiatric disorders in children is not as well documented as it is for adults. However, approximately 20% of children are estimated to have mental disorders with at least mild functional impairment. Children and adolescents with a serious emotional disturbance number approximately 5% to 9% of children ages 9 to 17 (New Freedom Commission on Mental Health, 2003).

Estimates suggest that approximately 20% of the older adult population have a diagnosable psychiatric disorder during a one-year period. This does not include cognitive impairments and dementias, the most common being Alzheimer's disease (New Freedom Commission on Mental Health, 2003).

Considerable research now documents that mental health is the key to overall physical health and well-being (Fawzy et al., 1993; Sephton et al., 2000). Compelling evidence reports that up to 75% of all primary care visits can be attributed to psychosocial problems, including mood, anxiety, and substance-related disorders (New Freedom Commission on Mental Health, 2003) and that mental health has a significant impact on clinical outcomes related to myocardial infarction, stroke (Whyte & Mulsant, 2002), cancer (Chochinov, 2001; Stark & House, 2000), and other chronic diseases like diabetes (deGroot et al., 2001).

Although the prevalence of psychiatric disorders did not significantly change between 1990–1992 (29.2%) and 2001–2003 (30.5%), the rate of treatment increased from 20.3% to 32.9% in the same period (Kessler et al., 2005), reflecting the expansion of primary care, managed care, and behavioral "carve-out" programs for mental health services. Note, however, that most people with psychiatric disorders still do not receive treatment for their disorder.

Disparities Among Diverse Populations

Data from the U.S. Census Bureau demonstrate significant changes in the racial and ethnic composition of the U.S. population. The percentage of non-Hispanic whites is projected to decrease from 70% in 2000 to 50% by 2050, with the greatest growth seen in Hispanic and Asian populations which are projected to double in the same period (U.S. Census Bureau, 2004). Although rates of mental illness in minority populations are estimated to be similar to those in the white population, minorities are less likely to receive mental health services and are likely to receive services of poorer quality (U.S. DHHS, 2001). Efforts to improve quality and access to mental health services for minority populations will include greater emphasis on developing cultural awareness and sensitivity among individual mental healthcare providers and increasing cultural competence in healthcare organizations. This will entail promotion of linguistic competence, including utilization of bilingual staff, more effective and widespread use of translation services, and redesign of written materials for persons with low English literacy.

Stigma and barriers to accessible, effective, and coordinated treatment contribute to health disparities within the population (Institute of Medicine, 2005). Financial barriers include lack of parity in insurance coverage for psychiatric-mental health care and treatment, resulting in restrictions on the number and type of outpatient visits and number of covered inpatient days, and high co-pays for services. Changes in eligibility criteria for public insurance programs have contributed to an increase in the number of uninsured. Reductions in reimbursement have affected the number of clinicians willing or able to afford to provide services at lower rates. Geographical barriers include lack of affordable, accessible public transportation in urban areas and lack of accessible clinical services in rural areas. Cultural issues, including lack of knowledge, fear, and stigma associated with mental illness, also constitute barriers to seeking help for mental health problems.

These disparities occur at a time of growing evidence regarding effective treatment of mental health problems and psychiatric disorders. Research evidence now supports the lifelong ability to influence the structure and function of the brain (brain plasticity) through manipulation of environmental, interpersonal, and behavioral factors. The evidence to support clinical decision-making by psychiatric nurses and other mental health professionals continues to accumulate.

Psychiatric-Mental Health Nursing Leadership in Transforming the Mental Health System

In the course of their practice, it is critical that psychiatric-mental health nurses consider the particular vision of mental health care that informs their practice. Federal agencies, commissions, and advocacy groups have identified a future vision of a mental healthcare system organized to respond to all consumers in need of services. These reports converge on several points, but most crucial is that a transformed mental health system is centered on the patient. Key to this vision are strategies for remedying the inadequacy and fragmentation of services and for creating a workforce to carry out the transformation. There is particular emphasis on providing services to children, adolescents, older adults, and other underserved populations. In leading the transformation of the mental healthcare delivery system, psychiatric-mental health nurses must understand the key threads in the government/agency/consumer group plan and the factors that can affect enactment.

Recovery is the lead principle of the transformation plans of the Substance Abuse and Mental Health Services Administration, National Alliance for the Mentally Ill, National Council on Disabilities, the Institute of Medicine, and the President's New Freedom Commission. The recovery paradigm of mental health care emphasizes reawakening of hope, engagement in life, and empowerment over illness. Recovery is a critical component of psychosocial rehabilitation, which also focuses on helping individuals develop the skills they need to assume meaningful employment, suitable housing, and interpersonal relationships (Anthony et al., 2002).

The person-centered recovery model supports an individualized and subjectively defined path to healing. It is an experience-based approach in which the process and outcome of recovery is defined and paced by the individual. In this era of evidence-based practice, intervention is driven by objective outcomes data derived scientifically to support prescriptive approaches. This creates a tension that must be explored and negotiated by psychiatric-mental health nurses; they must balance and integrate the science of evidence-based treatment with a philosophical understanding of how individuals attach meaning to experiences that shape their behavior and their treatment choices. With its grounding in the patient narrative, nursing is in an excellent position to maximize and integrate standard patient outcomes with desired outcomes defined by the patient (Raingruber, 1999; Barker, 2001; O'Brien, 2001; Raingruber, 2003; Forchuk et al., 2005; Salyers & Macy, 2005).

The transformation plan of the President's New Freedom Commission calls for community-level service systems that coordinate multiple agencies to provide care. These points of connection between agencies are vital to the realization of individualized recovery plans (SAMHSA, 2005). However, the notion of widespread outpatient community-based services runs contrary to the current trend of reduced funding for all forms of mental health treatment, including outpatient services (Manderscheid et al., 2004; Martin & Leslie, 2003; National Association of Psychiatric Health Systems, 2003).

A person with a serious and persistent psychiatric disorder may indeed move toward recovery with the assistance of interagency collaboration and assertive community treatment, but historically there has been no guarantee that the infrastructure would enact the plan (Phillips et al., 2001). A review of the past demonstrates that complex case management systems demand team leaders who are experienced, trained mental health professionals (Rapp, 1998), and that psychiatric nurses are a key agent for achieving positive patient outcomes in case management teams (McGrew & Bond, 1995).

The transformed mental health system will require nurses who understand systems and can work between and within systems, connecting services and acting as an important safety net in the event of service gaps. Psychiatric nurses are perfectly positioned to fill this role and make significant contributions to positive clinical recovery outcomes for the vulnerable, and often underserved, patient population.

The mental health transformation plan in the President's New Freedom Commission Report also calls for inclusion of the homeless, children, older adults, rural sector, and other underserved populations. Certainly an ideology of inclusion restores both equity and humanity to the system. But for many of these groups social problems are inextricably bound with emotional illness.

A recent study of children with serious emotional disorder (SED) found that almost half had social, family, and educational issues as well (Pottick et al., 2002). Evidence related to psychiatric disorders in older adults reveals high rates of co-morbid medical illness. Co-morbidity in the aged is a predictor of poorer response to mental health treatment, as well as a predictor of relapse (Hanrahan & Sullivan-Marx, 2005). Moreover, despite a dramatic growth in evidence-based treatment for mental health problems in older adults, mental health service use is extremely low. Less than 3% of older adults receive outpatient mental health services, only 7% inpatient psychiatric services, and 9% private psychiatric care (Persky, 1998).

Nursing models for rural care are specifically designed to address the interplay of poverty, mental illness, and social issues (Hauenstein, 1997). Such nursing models recognize that resource-poor environments require service models with provisions for moving clients into self-management and for bridging systems so that medical issues are addressed. This nursing approach will be of significant importance in crafting individualized treatment plans for populations with tremendous physical and social needs inextricably bound with their mental health issues. The need for psychiatric nurses will be great because their command of multiple bodies of knowledge (medical science, neurobiology of psychiatric disorders, treatment methods, and relationship science) positions them as the healthcare professionals best suited to maintain the connection between psychiatry, medicine, and case management systems (Hanrahan & Sullivan-Marx, 2005).

Prevention

Psychiatric-mental health nurses also lead prevention efforts. Armed with the growing understanding of how stress and mental illness interact, psychiatric-mental health nurses educate the public on the ramifications of stress and om stress reduction techniques (deVries & Wilkerson, 2003). Increasingly, researchers are demonstrating the promise of prevention via intervention into sub-threshold symptoms (Kuijpers, Van Straten, & Smit, 2005). Nursing's traditional focus on primary prevention will fit nicely with this effort to treat mental conditions in early stages. The behaviors that place youth at risk are priority foci for prevention efforts.

While traditional prevention foci (such as decreasing tobacco, alcohol, and substance use) continue, increased attention is being directed to the effects of media and the Internet on teens' risk behaviors. Though youth spend, on average, three hours a day watching television and spend two hours online at least four times a week, little is known about how this media saturation shapes their normative behaviors and social interaction patterns (Escobar-Chaves et al., 2005). Depression in adolescence is an important focus for early identification and intervention (Draucker, 2005). School nurses, often the first contact with youth, already function as key mental health service providers, and their role in prevention should be strengthened and supported by the specialty.

The Evolving Role of National Data Systems to Improve Quality

Another key to the transformed mental healthcare system is consumer input in determining the indicators used to gauge quality. The government is seeking to define and capture quality on the patient level via the development of an information system, termed the DS2000 (Duffy et al., 2004). This system exemplifies the broad use of information technology to capture not just quality data but provider data, cost, and outcomes. With its full implementation, decision support would link quality performance to quality outcomes and payment information. The hope is to establish a large data system that providers, mental health systems, and state planners could access to determine what works, at what cost, with what type of patient.

Quality initiatives should be implemented in an integrated fashion, whereby clinicians are accountable for understanding and using technology to build an evidence base for their practice. As clinicians, psychiatric nurses must understand that technology is the vehicle for data accountability that will be used to gauge quality of care and to revise policy. Psychiatric nursing faculty members are in an excellent position to use technology in the educational process and thus create future clinicians who are fluent in its use (Carlson-Sabelli & Delaney, 2005; McGuiness & Noonan, 2004).

Evidence-Based Practice and Lifelong Learning

The transformed mental healthcare system will require a mental health workforce with additional characteristics. It is a workforce that must be comfortable with the use of technology in care delivery, able to operate in teams, and fluent in the use of evidence-based practice (Stuart, Tondora, & Hoge, 2004).

The transition to evidence-based practice has been rapid and not without its critics (Norcross, Beutler, & Levant, 2005). The use of the "best available" research evidence, coupled with expert clinical judgment and patient preferences, creates essential linkages among the patient, the provider, the setting, and the science (Sackett, 2000). The key is that the person is not relegated to either extreme—being a patient or a consumer—and that evidence-based practices are always maintained in a relationship-based approach (Messer, 2006).

Advances in genetics and innovative treatments for major mental illness are the promise of the future (Kestenbaum, 2000). Psychiatric disorders occur as the result of complex interactions between genes, behavior, personality, and the environment. Estimates of genetic risk for psychiatric disorders are the outcomes of population studies, twin studies, adoption studies, first- and second-degree relatives (pedigree) studies, neuroimaging studies, and molecular linkage studies. Gene mapping involves the study of the interaction of multiple abnormal genes that augment vulnerability to a specific psychiatric disorder (Pestka, 2003; Sapolsky, 2003). An earlier age of onset increases the likelihood of inheritability in selected disorders such as Alzheimer's disease.

Environmental factors and behavior influence the expression of the inheritable psychiatric disorders. Major stressful events such as an insult to the brain during fetal development, stress and trauma, medical illness, and illicit drug use can raise the risk for symptoms of the disorder to begin. Identification of and education about risk factors and strategies for lifestyle modifications is warranted when there is a high-risk family history. Pharmacogenetics, which matches DNA variants such as fast or slow metabolizers to individualized pharmacological treatments, holds promise. Gene expression, gene therapy, and vaccines to alter genetic expression are future tools to prevent or treat certain disorders.

Psychiatric nursing leads in creating client-centered care based on the evidence related to the neurobiology of psychiatric disorders and the effects of medications, but it also constructs relationships within a recovery-based model (Forchuk et al., 2005). This demands a commitment to continuing professional development, lifelong learning, and a working knowledge of the current literature.

Safety for Patients and for PMH Nurses

While the transformed mental healthcare system is largely dedicated to the creation of new service structures, none of the agencies have lost sight of safety (Spear, 2005). Especially pertinent to nursing practice are safety issues surrounding restraint and information that error and mortality rates can be tied to nurse–patient ratios. As scrutiny of safety and errors continues, nurses have assumed key roles in designing studies on the relationship of nursing, staffing, and patient safety. They must also maintain roles consistent with their direct care position, anticipate systems errors, and employ preventive safety measures. In the inpatient arena, psychiatric nurses, as managers of the milieu, must move the safety agenda beyond reducing restraint to a studied approach of how to create safe units, both physical and psychological, and develop, measure, and evaluate key systems and staffing factors that result in reductions in restraint, violence, and other threats to patient safety (Johnson & Delaney, 2006; Delaney, 2005).

Definition of Psychiatric-Mental Health Nursing

Nursing's Social Policy Statement (ANA, 2003) defines nursing as "the protection, promotion, and optimization of health and abilities, prevention of illness and injury, alleviation of suffering through the diagnosis and treatment of human response, and advocacy in the care of individuals, families, communities, and populations."

Psychiatric-mental health nursing is a specialized area of nursing practice committed to promoting mental health through the assessment, diagnosis, and treatment of human responses to mental health problems and psychiatric disorders. Psychiatric-mental health nursing, a core mental health profession, employs a purposeful use of self as its art and a wide range of nursing, psychosocial, and neurobiological theories and research evidence as its science. Psychiatric-mental health nurses provide comprehensive, patient-centered mental health and psychiatric care in a variety of settings across the continuum of care. Essential components of this specialty practice include health and wellness promotion through identification of mental health issues, prevention of mental health problems, care of mental health problems, and treatment of persons with psychiatric disorders.

It is within the scope of psychiatric-mental health nursing practice to provide mental health care to patients seeking mental health services in a wide range of delivery settings. Mental health care involves overall health promotion, universal, selective, and preventive interventions (Mrazek & Hagerty, 1994), general health teaching, health screening and appropriate referral for treatment of general or complex health problems, and a specialization in the evaluation and management of those with psychiatric disorders and those at risk for them, including psychiatric rehabilitation (Haber & Billings, 1995).

The psychiatric nurse's assessment synthesizes information obtained from interviews, behavioral observations, and other available data. From these, the psychiatric nurse determines diagnoses or problem statements that are congruent with available and accepted classification systems and develops a treatment plan based on assessment data and theoretical premises. The nurse then selects and implements interventions and periodically evaluates patient outcomes, revising the plan of care as needed, to achieve optimal results. Use of standardized classification systems enhances communication and permits the data to be used for research.

Mental health problems and psychiatric disorders are addressed across a continuum of care. A continuum of care consists of an integrated system of settings, services, healthcare clinicians, and care levels spanning states from illness to wellness. The primary goal of a continuum of care is to provide treatment that allows the patient to achieve the highest level of functioning in the least restrictive environment.

Psychiatric-mental health advanced practice nursing involves the delivery of comprehensive primary mental health care in a variety of settings. Primary mental health care is defined as the continuous and comprehensive services necessary for the promotion of optimal health; the prevention of mental illness; health maintenance; management of, and referral for, mental and physical health problems; the diagnosis and treatment of psychiatric disorders and their sequelae, and rehabilitation (Haber & Billings, 1995). Psychiatric-mental health nursing is necessarily holistic and considers the needs and strengths of the individual, family, group, and community.

Phenomena of Concern for Psychiatric-Mental Health Nurses

Phenomena of concern for psychiatric-mental health nurses include:

- Promotion of optimal mental and physical health and well-being and prevention of mental illness.
- Impaired ability to function related to psychiatric, emotional, and physiological distress.
- Alterations in thinking, perceiving, and communicating due to psychiatric disorders or mental health problems.
- Behaviors and mental states that indicate potential danger to self or others.
- Emotional stress related to illness, pain, disability, and loss.
- Symptom management, side effects or toxicities associated with self-administered drugs, psychopharmological intervention, and other treatment modalities.
- The barriers to treatment efficacy and recovery posed by alcohol and substance abuse and dependence.
- Self-concept and body image changes, developmental issues, life process changes, and end-of-life issues.
- Physical symptoms that occur along with altered psychological status.

- Psychological symptoms that occur along with altered physiological status.

- Interpersonal, organizational, sociocultural, spiritual, or environmental circumstances or events which have an effect on the mental and emotional well-being of the individual and family or community.

- Elements of recovery, including the ability to maintain housing, employment, and social support, that help individuals re-engage in seeking meaningful lives.

- Societal factors such as violence, poverty, and substance abuse.

Levels of Psychiatric-Mental Health Nursing Practice

Psychiatric-mental health nurses are registered nurses who are educationally prepared in nursing and licensed to practice in their individual states. Levels of practice are differentiated by educational preparation, complexity of practice, and performance of certain nursing functions (SERPN, 2005).

Psychiatric-Mental Health Registered Nurse (RN-PMH)

A Psychiatric-Mental Health Registered Nurse (RN-PMH) is a registered nurse who demonstrates competence, including specialized knowledge, skills, and abilities, obtained through education and experience in caring for persons with mental health issues, mental health problems, and psychiatric disorders.

Nurses from a number of educational backgrounds participate and practice in psychiatric nursing settings. Due to the complexity of care in the specialty, the preferred educational preparation is at the baccalaureate level with credentialing by the American Nurses Credentialing Center (ANCC).

The science of nursing is based on a critical thinking framework, known as the nursing process, composed of assessment, diagnosis, outcomes identification, planning, implementation, and evaluation. These steps serve as the foundation for clinical decision-making and are used to provide an evidence base for practice (ANA, 2004).

Psychiatric-mental health registered nursing practice is characterized by the use of the nursing process to treat people with actual or potential mental health problems or psychiatric disorders to: promote and foster health and safety; assess dysfunction; assist persons to regain or improve their coping abilities; maximize strengths; and prevent further disability. Data collection at the point of contact involves observational and investigative activities, which are guided by the nurse's knowledge of human behavior and the principles of the psychiatric interviewing process.

The data may include but is not limited to the patient's:

- Central complaint, focus, or concern and symptoms of major psychiatric disorders.

- History and presentation regarding suicidal, violent, and self-mutilating behaviors.

- History of reliability with regard to patient's verbal agreement to seek professional assistance before engaging in behaviors dangerous to self or others.

- Pertinent family history of psychiatric disorders, substance abuse, and other mental and relevant physical health issues.

- Evidence of abuse, neglect, or trauma.

- Stressors, contributing factors, and coping strategies.

- Demographic profile and history of health patterns, illnesses, past treatments, and level of adherence and effectiveness of those in treatment.

- Actual or potential barriers to adherence to recommended or prescribed treatment.

- Health beliefs and practices.

- Method of communication.

- Religious and spiritual beliefs and practices.

- Cultural, racial, and ethnic identity and practices.

- Physical, developmental, cognitive, mental status, emotional health concerns, and neurological assessment.

- Daily activities, personal hygiene, occupational functioning, functional health status, and social roles.

- Work, sleep, and sexual functioning.

- Economic, political, legal, and environmental factors affecting health.

- Significant support systems and community resources, including those that have been available and underutilized.

- Knowledge, satisfaction, and motivation to change, related to health.

- Strengths and competencies that can be used to promote health.

- Current and past medications, both prescribed and over-the-counter, including herbs, alternative medications, vitamins, or nutritional supplements.

- Medication interactions and history of side effects and past efficacy.

- Allergies and other adverse reactions.

- History and patterns of alcohol and substance abuse, including type, amount, most recent use, and withdrawal symptoms.

- Complementary therapies used to treat health and mental illness and their outcomes.

The work of psychiatric-mental health registered nurses is accomplished through the nurse–client relationship, therapeutic intervention skills, and professional attributes. These attributes include but are not limited to self awareness, empathy, and moral integrity, which enable psychiatric-mental health nurses to practice the artful use of self in therapeutic relationships. Some characteristics of artful therapeutic practice are respect for the client, availability, spontaneity, hope, acceptance, sensitivity, vision, accountability, advocacy, and spirituality.

Psychiatric-mental health registered nurses practice in a variety of clinical settings across the care continuum and engage in a broad array of clinical activities including, but not limited to, health promotion and health maintenance; intake screening, evaluation, and triage; case management; provision of therapeutic and safe environments; promotion of self-care activities; administration of psychobiological treatment regimens and monitoring response and effects; crisis intervention and stabilization; and psychiatric rehabilitation.

Psychiatric-mental health registered nurses play a significant role in the articulation and implementation of new paradigms of care and treatment that place the patient at the center of the care delivery system. They are key members of interdisciplinary teams in implementing initiatives such as seclusion and restraint reduction or elimination, patient involvement in treatment planning processes, and skill-building programs to assist patients to achieve their own goals.

Psychiatric-mental health registered nurses maintain current knowledge of advances in genetics and neuroscience and their impact on psychopharmocology and other treatment modalities. In partnership with patients, communities, and other health professionals, psychiatric-mental health nurses provide leadership in identifying mental health issues, and in developing strategies to ameliorate or prevent them.

Psychiatric-Mental Health Advanced Practice Registered Nurse (APRN-PMH)

The Psychiatric-Mental Health Advanced Practice Registered Nurse (APRN-PMH) is a licensed registered nurse who is educationally prepared at the master's or doctorate level in the specialty of psychiatric-mental health nursing and holds advanced practice specialty certification from ANCC. The APRN-PMH expands the practice of a registered nurse by demonstrating a greater depth and breadth of knowledge, a greater synthesis of data, increased complexity of skills and interventions, and significant role autonomy (ANA, 2004).

The American Nurses Association (ANA) defines Advanced Practice Registered Nurses (APRNs) as professional nurses who have successfully completed a graduate program of study in a nursing specialty that provides specialized knowledge and skills that form the foundation for expanded roles in health care.

The full scope and standards of practice for psychiatric-mental health advanced practice nursing are set forth in this document. While individual APRN-PMHs may actually implement portions of the full scope and practice based on their role, position description, and practice setting, it is, importantly, the full breadth of the knowledge base that informs their practice.

APRN-PMH practice focuses on the application of competencies, knowledge, and experience to individuals, families, or groups with complex psychiatric-mental health problems. Promoting mental health in society is a significant role for the APRN-PMH, as is collaboration with and referral to other health professionals as either the patient's need or the APRN-PMH's practice focus may dictate.

The scope of practice in psychiatric-mental health nursing is continually expanding as the context of practice, the need for patient access to holistic care, and the various scientific and nursing knowledge bases evolve. It is within the scope of practice of the APRN-PMH to provide primary mental health care to patients seeking mental health services in a wide range of delivery settings. APRN-PMHs are accountable for functioning within the parameters of their education and training, and the scope of practice as defined by their state practice acts. APRN-PMHs are responsible for making referrals for health problems that are outside their scope of practice. Although many primary care clinicians treat some symptoms of mental health problems and psychiatric disorders, the APRN-PMH provides a full range of comprehensive services that constitute primary mental health and psychiatric care and treatment.

APRN-PMHs are professionally qualified to assume responsibility for clinical functions. They are accountable for their own practice and are prepared to perform services independent of other disciplines in the full range of delivery settings. The educational preparation of advanced practice psychiatric-mental health nurses in both the biological and social sciences gives them a unique ability to differentiate various aspects of the patient's functioning and to make appropriate judgments and decisions about the need for interventions, referral, or consultation with other clinicians (ANA, 2004).

Additional functions of the APRN-PMH include prescribing psychopharmacological agents, integrative therapy interventions, various forms of psychotherapy, community interventions, case management, consultation and liaison, clinical supervision, expanded advocacy activities, education, and research.

Psychotherapy

Psychotherapy interventions include all generally accepted methods of brief or long-term therapy, specifically including individual therapy, group therapy, marital or couple therapy, and family therapy using a range of therapy models including, but not limited to, insight-oriented, cognitive, behavioral, and interpersonal therapies to produce change or supportive therapy to maintain function.

Psychotherapy denotes a formally structured relationship between the therapist (APRN-PMH) and the patient for the explicit purpose of effecting negotiated outcomes. This treatment approach to mental disorders is intended to alleviate emotional distress or symptoms, to reverse or change maladaptive behaviors, and to facilitate personal growth and development. The contract with the patient or client is usually verbal but may be written. It includes well accepted elements such as purpose of the therapy, time, place, fees, confidentiality and privacy provisions, and emergency after-hours contact information.

Psychopharmacological Interventions

Psychopharmacological interventions include the prescribing or recommending of pharmacologic agents and the ordering and interpretation of diagnostic and laboratory testing. In utilizing any psychobiological intervention, including the prescribing of psychoactive medications, the APRN-PMH intentionally seeks specific therapeutic responses, anticipates common side effects, safeguards against adverse drug interactions, and is alert for unintended or toxic responses.

Case Management

Case management by the APRN-PMH involves population-specific nursing knowledge coupled with research, knowledge of the social and legal systems related to mental health, and expertise to engage a wide range of services for the patient, regardless of setting. The APRN-PMH may oversee or directly engage in case management activities. The APRN-PMH analyzes barriers to care and intervenes to change or improve systems to mobilize therapeutic resources needed by the patient for optimum outcomes. Case management activities may be with a single client or with a designated population such as the seriously and persistently mentally ill.

Program Development and Management

In the community, the APRN-PMH may focus on the mental health needs of the population as a whole. The APRN-PMH may design programs to meet the mental health needs of a population (such as the seriously and persistently mentally ill) or to target a population at risk for developing mental health problems through health and wellness promotion, identification and amelioration of risk factors, screening, and early intervention. These activities are informed by the full range of nursing knowledge which includes a holistic approach to individuals, families, and communities that is cognizant and respectful of cultural and spiritual norms and values.

Consultation and Liaison

Consultation and liaison activities take place in general (non-psychiatric) healthcare arenas such as hospitals, extended care facilities, rehabilitation centers, schools, nursing homes, and outpatient clinics. The consultation and liaison role of the psychiatric-mental health nurse centers on providing mental health specialist consultation or direct care psychiatric-mental health nursing services.

The clinical aspect of the role ranges from mental health promotion to illness rehabilitation. In consultation and liaison activities, the APRN-PMH concentrates on the emotional, spiritual, developmental, cognitive, and behavioral responses of patients who enter any setting of the healthcare system with actual or potential physiological dysfunction (patient-centered consultation). The psychiatric-mental health consultation may include consultee-centered consultation with nurses and clinicians in other specialty areas to increase their biopsychosocial knowledge and skills. Such consultation may also assist consultees to recognize and manage their own reactions to patients that could adversely affect their patient care if undetected and unaddressed. Psychiatric-mental health consultation may also include assessment and recommendations for action when the healthcare delivery organization is the client (administrative consultation) (Caplan & Caplan, 1993).

Clinical Supervision

The APRN-PMH provides clinical supervision to assist other mental health clinicians to expand their clinical practice skills, to meet the standard requirement for ongoing peer consultation, and for essential peer supervision. This process is aimed at professional growth and development rather than staff performance evaluation. Through education, preparation, and clinical experience, the APRN-PMH is qualified to provide clinical supervision at the request of other mental health clinicians and clinician-trainees. As a clinical supervisor, the APRN-PMH is expected both to be involved in direct patient care and to serve as a clinical role model and a clinical consultant.

APRN-PMH nurses providing clinical supervision must be aware of the potential for impaired professional objectivity or exploitation when they have dual or multiple relationships with the supervisee or patients. The nurse should avoid providing clinical supervision for people with whom they have pre-existing relationships that could hinder objectivity. Nurses who provide clinical supervision maintain the confidentiality of staff and patients, except as is required for evaluation and necessary reporting.

Ethical Issues in Psychiatric-Mental Health Nursing

Psychiatric-mental health registered nurses adhere to all aspects of *Code of Ethics for Nurses with Interpretive Statements* (ANA, 2001). The psychiatric-mental health registered nurse monitors and carefully manages therapeutic self-disclosure. The nurse demonstrates a commitment to practicing self-care, managing stress, nurturing self, and maintaining supportive relationships with others so that the nurse is meeting their own needs outside of the therapeutic relationship. The psychiatric-mental health registered nurse is always cognizant of the responsibility to balance patient rights with patient safety and the potential need for coercive practices (e.g., restrictive measures such as restraint or seclusion), or forced treatment (e.g., court-mandated treatment, mental hygiene arrest for an emergent psychiatric evaluation) when the patient lacks the ability to maintain their own safety. The psychiatric-mental health registered nurse helps resolve ethical issues of patients, colleagues, or systems as evidenced in such activities as consulting with and serving on ethics committees.

Specialized Areas of Practice

Specialty programs in psychiatric-mental health nursing generally focus on adult or child-adolescent psychiatric-mental health nursing, and certifications are currently available for these two specialties. Areas of focus within psychiatric-mental health nursing have emerged based on current and anticipated societal needs. These areas may be organized according to a developmental period (geriatric), a specific mental or emotional disorder (depression, severe and persistent mental illness, developmental disability), a particular practice focus (forensics, addictions, community, family, couple, individual), or a specific role or function (case management, consultation and liaison).

Psychiatric-Mental Health Nursing Clinical Practice Settings

The settings and arrangements for psychiatric-mental health nursing practice vary widely in purpose, type, and location, and in the auspices under which they are operated. Psychiatric-mental health nurses may work in organized settings and may be paid for their services on a salaried, contractual, or fee-for-service basis. In addition, the APRN-PMH may be self-employed or employed by an agency, practice autonomously or collaboratively, and bill clients for services provided.

Today, because of the advances in brain research and pharmacological treatments, as well as the current focus on cost-effective treatment, most clients in need of mental health services are cared for in community settings. Acute, intermediate, and long-term care settings still admit and care for psychiatric patients but lengths of stay, especially in acute and intermediate settings, have decreased in response to fiscal mandates, the availability of community-based settings, and consumer preference.

Crisis Intervention and Psychiatric Emergency Services

Crisis intervention units may be found in the emergency department of a general or psychiatric hospital or within centers in the community. Patients in crisis demonstrate severe symptoms and require a high intensity of nursing services.

Acute Inpatient Care

This setting involves the most intensive care and is reserved for acutely ill patients who are at high risk for harming themselves or others, or are unable to care for their basic needs. This treatment is often short-term. These units may be in a psychiatric hospital, a general hospital, or a publicly funded psychiatric facility or program.

Intermediate and Long-Term Care

Intermediate and long-term care facilities may admit patients but more often they receive patients transferred from acute care settings. Intermediate and long-term care provides treatment and rehabilitation for patients who are at chronic risk for harming themselves or others due to mental illness. Long-term inpatient care usually involves a minimum of three months. Both public and private psychiatric facilities provide this type of care.

Partial Hospitalization and Intensive Outpatient Treatment

The aim of partial hospitalization and intensive outpatient programs is acute symptom stabilization for patients with safe housing options or employment. Partial hospitalization may also serve as a step down for patients discharged from an inpatient unit.

Residential Services

A residential facility provides care for patients over a twenty-four-hour period. Services in typical residential treatment facilities include psycho-education around symptom management and medications, assistance with vocational training, and, in the case of the severely and persistently mentally ill, may include training for activities of daily living. Rehabilita-tion is often a goal for residential treatment facilities.

Community-Based Care

Psychiatric-mental health registered nurses provide care within the com-munity as an effective method of responding to the mental health needs of individuals, families, and groups. Community-based care refers to care delivered in partnership with patients in their homes, work sites, mental health clinics and programs, health maintenance organizations, shelters and clinics for the homeless, crisis centers, senior centers, group homes, and other community settings. Schools and colleges are important sites of mental health promotion, primary prevention, and early intervention programs for children and youth that involve psychiatric-mental health registered nurses. Psychiatric-mental health registered nurses are involved in educating teachers, parents, and students about mental health issues and in efforts such as depression screening. They may also provide mental health assessments and psychiatric services to students.

Assertive Community Treatment (ACT)

The Assertive Community Treatment model is an interdisciplinary team approach to the care of people with severe mental illness; it provides services in the individual's natural setting, including homeless shelters. ACT provides a comprehensive range of treatments. The goals of ACT are to help patients meet the requirements of community living after discharge from another more restricted form of care, and to reduce re-currences of hospitalization.

Primary Care

Because of recent changes in the healthcare system, primary care set-tings have assumed increasing importance in treating mental disorders.

Depression is now more likely to be treated in primary care than in specialty mental health settings (Olfson et al., 2002). Psychiatric-mental health registered nurses provide mental health services in primary care via several models:

- consultation: the APRN-PMH functions as an expert resource for primary care providers;
- provision: patients are referred to an APRN-PMH affiliated with the primary care setting;
- integrated: APRN-PMHs who have additional training in primary care provide a mixture of psychiatric and primary care services; and
- collaborative: a network of primary care and mental health providers collaboratively manage a group of patients.

Psychiatric-mental health nurses at both the RN and APRN level participate in large-scale initiatives to improve the quality of depression care in primary care settings (Koike, Unutzer, & Wells, 2002).

Integrative Programs

Integrative programs provide simultaneous care for co-occurring substance use disorders and serious mental health disorders by a team of trained professionals. Services include assertive outreach, comprehensive services, and shared decision-making with staff, patients, and patients' families. Treatment progresses in stages from engagement in treatment to relapse prevention, incorporating a long-term commitment to services and pharmacological interventions. Sustained remission rates from substance use, lower rates of victimization, longer retention in treatment, and less time in the hospital are outcomes of integrated treatment for co-occurring disorders. Levels of care are determined by the severity of the substance use disorder and the severity of the mental illness. Those with the most severe disorders may be treated in specialized residential treatment centers or modified therapeutic communities.

Telehealth

Telehealth is the use of telecommunications technology to remove time and distance barriers from the delivery of healthcare services and related healthcare activities. It is an expanded means of communication that promotes access to health care. The psychiatric-mental health registered nurse may use electronic means of communication such as telephone consultation, computers, electronic mail, image transmission, and interactive video sessions to establish and maintain a therapeutic relationship with patients by creating an alternative sense of the nursing presence that may or may not occur in "real time". Psychiatric-mental health nursing care in telehealth incorporates practice and clinical guidelines that are based on empirical evidence and professional consensus. Telehealth encounters raise special issues related to confidentiality and regulation. Telehealth technology can cross state and even national boundaries and must be practiced in accordance with all applicable state, federal, and international laws and regulations. Particular attention must be directed to confidentiality, informed consent, documentation, maintenance of records, and the integrity of the transmitted information.

Self-Employment

Self-employed psychiatric-mental health advanced practice nurses offer direct services in solo private practice and group practice settings, or through contracts with employee assistance programs, health maintenance organizations, managed care companies, preferred provider organizations, industry health departments, home healthcare agencies, or other service delivery arrangements. In these settings, the APRN-PMH provides primary mental health care to clients in the nurse's caseload. In the consultation and liaison role, the APRN-PMH may also contract for consultation services directed at either the needs of the organization and its staff or the needs of patients in a variety of healthcare settings (nursing homes, medical units, home health care). Self-employed nurses may also form nurse-owned corporations or organizations that would provide mental health service contracts to industries or employers.

Forensic Mental Health

Recent studies have noted the high rates of mental illness in jails and prisons. APRN-PMHs perform psychiatric assessments, prescribe and administer psychiatric medications, and educate correctional officers about mental health issues. They are also involved in providing therapeutic services to witnesses or victims of crime.

Disaster Mental Health

Psychiatric-mental health nurses provide psychological first aid and mental health clinical services as first responders through organizational systems in response to environmental and man-made disasters.

STANDARDS OF PRACTICE

The following Standards of Practice and Standards of Professional Performance are written in such a way that each standard and its measurement criteria listed for the Psychiatric-Mental Health Registered Nurse also apply to the Advanced Practice Psychiatric-Mental Health Registered Nurse. In several instances additional standards and measurement criteria for the APRN-PMH are only applicable to the Advanced Practice Registered Nurse.

STANDARD 1. ASSESSMENT
The Psychiatric-Mental Health Registered Nurse collects comprehensive health data that is pertinent to the patient's health or situation.

Measurement Criteria

The Psychiatric-Mental Health Registered Nurse (PRN-PMH):

- Collects data in a systematic and ongoing process.

- Involves the patient, family, other healthcare providers, and others in the patient's environment, as appropriate, in holistic data collection.

- Demonstrates effective clinical interviewing skills that facilitate development of a therapeutic alliance.

- Prioritizes data collection activities based on the patient's immediate condition or anticipated needs of the patient or situation.

- Uses appropriate evidence-based assessment techniques and instruments in collecting pertinent data.

- Uses analytical models and problem-solving techniques.

- Ensures that appropriate consents, as determined by regulations and policies, are obtained to protect patient confidentiality and support the patient's rights in the process of data gathering.

- Synthesizes available data, information, and knowledge relevant to the situation to identify patterns and variances.

Continued ▶

- Uses therapeutic principles to understand and make inferences about the patient's emotions, thoughts, and behaviors.

- Documents relevant data in a retrievable format.

Additional Measurement Criteria for the Psychiatric-Mental Health Advanced Practice Registered Nurse

The APRN-PMH:

- Employs evidence-based clinical practice guidelines to guide screening and diagnostic activities as available and appropriate.

- Performs a comprehensive psychiatric and mental health evaluation.

- Initiates and interprets diagnostic tests and procedures relevant to the patient's current status.

- Conducts a multigenerational family assessment, including medical and psychiatric history.

- Assesses interactions among the individual, family, community, and social systems and their relationship to mental health functioning.

STANDARD 2. DIAGNOSIS
The Psychiatric-Mental Health Registered Nurse analyzes the assessment data to determine diagnoses or problems, including level of risk.

Measurement Criteria

The Psychiatric-Mental Health Registered Nurse (RN-PMH):

- Identifies actual or potential risks to the patient's health and safety or barriers to mental and physical health which may include but are not limited to interpersonal, systematic, or environmental circumstances.

- Derives the diagnosis or problems from the assessment data.

- Validates the diagnosis or problems with the patient, significant others, and other healthcare clinicians when possible and appropriate.

- Develops diagnoses or problem statements that are congruent with available and accepted classification systems.

- Documents diagnoses or problems in a manner that facilitates the determination of the expected outcomes and plan.

Additional Measurement Criteria for the Psychiatric-Mental Health Advanced Practice Registered Nurse

The APRN-PMH:

- Systematically compares and contrasts clinical findings with normal and abnormal variations and developmental events in formulating a differential diagnosis.

- Utilizes complex data and information obtained during interview, examination, and diagnostic procedures in identifying diagnosis.

- Identifies long-term effects of psychiatric disorders on mental, physical, and social health.

- Evaluates the health impact of life stressors, traumatic events, and situational crises within the context of the family cycle.

- Evaluates the impact of the course of psychiatric disorders and mental health problems on quality of life and functional status.

- Assists staff in developing and maintaining competency in the diagnostic process.

STANDARD 3. OUTCOMES IDENTIFICATION
The Psychiatric-Mental Health Registered Nurse identifies expected outcomes for a plan individualized to the patient or to the situation.

Measurement Criteria

The Psychiatric-Mental Health Registered Nurse (RN-PMH):

- Derives culturally appropriate expected outcomes from the diagnosis.

- Involves the patient, family, and other healthcare providers in formulating expected outcomes when possible and appropriate.

- Considers associated risks, benefits, costs, current scientific evidence, and clinical expertise when formulating expected outcomes.

- Defines expected outcomes in terms of the patient, patient values, ethical considerations, environment, or situation with consideration of associated risks, benefits, costs, and current scientific evidence.

- Develops expected outcomes that provide direction for continuity of care.

- Documents expected outcomes as measurable goals.

- Includes a time estimate for attainment of expected outcomes.

- Modifies expected outcomes based on changes in the status of the patient or evaluation of the situation.

Additional Measurement Criteria for the Psychiatric-Mental Health Advanced Practice Registered Nurse

The APRN-PMH:

- Identifies expected outcomes that incorporate scientific evidence and are achievable through implementation of evidence-based practices.

- Identifies expected outcomes that incorporate cost and clinical effectiveness, patient satisfaction, and continuity and consistency among providers.

- Supports and uses clinical guidelines linked to positive patient outcomes.

STANDARD 4. PLANNING
The Psychiatric-Mental Health Registered Nurse develops a plan that prescribes strategies and alternatives to attain expected outcomes.

Measurement Criteria

The Psychiatric-Mental Health Registered Nurse (RN-PMH):

- Develops an individualized plan considering patient characteristics or the situation.
- Develops the plan in collaboration with the patient, family, and other healthcare providers when appropriate.
- Considers the economic impact of the plan.
- Prioritizes elements of the plan based on the assessment of the patient's level of risk for potential harm to self or others and safety needs.
- Establishes the plan priorities with the patient, family, and others as appropriate.
- Includes strategies in the plan that address each of the identified diagnoses or issues, which may include strategies for promotion and restoration of health and prevention of illness, injury, and disease.
- Assists patients in securing treatment or services in the least restrictive environment.
- Includes an implementation pathway or timeline in the plan.
- Provides for continuity in the plan.
- Utilizes the plan to provide direction to other members of the healthcare team.
- Documents the plan using standardized language or recognized terminology.
- Defines the plan to reflect current statutes, rules and regulations, and standards.
- Utilizes current available research in planning care.
- Modifies the plan based on ongoing assessment of the patient's response and other outcome indicators.

Continued ▶

Additional Measurement Criteria for the Psychiatric-Mental Health Advanced Practice Registered Nurse

The APRN-PMH:

- Identifies assessment and diagnostic strategies and therapeutic interventions that reflect current evidence, including data, research, literature, and expert clinical knowledge.

- Plans care to minimize complications and promote function and quality of life using treatment modalities such as, but not limited to, behavioral therapies, psychotherapy, and psychopharmacology.

- Selects or designs strategies to meet the multifaceted needs of complex patients.

- Includes synthesis of patients' values and beliefs regarding nursing and medical therapies in the plan.

STANDARD 5. IMPLEMENTATION
The Psychiatric-Mental Health Registered Nurse implements the identified plan.

Measurement Criteria

The Psychiatric-Mental Health Registered Nurse (RN-PMH):

- Implements the plan in a safe and timely manner.

- Documents implementation and any modifications, including changes or omissions, of the identified plan.

- Utilizes evidence-based interventions and treatments specific to the diagnosis or problem.

- Provides age-appropriate care in a culturally and ethnically sensitive manner.

- Utilizes community resources and systems to implement the plan.

- Collaborates with nursing colleagues and others to implement the plan.

- Manages psychiatric emergencies by determining the level of risk and initiating and coordinating effective emergency care.

Additional Measurement Criteria for the Psychiatric-Mental Health Advanced Practice Registered Nurse

The APRN-PMH:

- Facilitates utilization of systems and community resources to implement the plan.

- Supports collaboration with nursing colleagues and other disciplines to implement the plan.

- Incorporates new knowledge and strategies to initiate change in nursing care practices if desired outcomes are not achieved.

- Uses principles and concepts of project management and systems management when implementing the plan.

- Fosters organizational systems that support implementation of the plan.

STANDARD 5A. COORDINATION OF CARE
The Psychiatric-Mental Health Registered Nurse coordinates care delivery.

Measurement Criteria

The Psychiatric-Mental Health Registered Nurse (RN-PMH):

- Coordinates implementation of the plan.

- Documents the coordination of care.

Additional Measurement Criteria for the Psychiatric-Mental Health Advanced Practice Registered Nurse

The APRN-PMH:

- Provides leadership in the coordination of multidisciplinary health care for integrated delivery of patient care services.

- Synthesizes data and information to prescribe necessary system and community support measures, including environmental modifications.

- Coordinates system and community resources that enhance delivery of care across continuums.

- Assists patients in getting financial assistance as needed to maintain appropriate care

STANDARD 5B. HEALTH TEACHING AND HEALTH PROMOTION
The Psychiatric-Mental Health Registered Nurse employs strategies to promote health and a safe environment.

Measurement Criteria

The Psychiatric-Mental Health Registered Nurse (RN-PMH):

- Uses health promotion and health teaching methods appropriate to the situation, patient's developmental level, learning needs, readiness, ability to learn, language preference, and culture.

- Provides health teaching related to the patient's needs and situation that may include, but is not limited to, mental health problems and psychiatric disorders, treatment regimen, coping skills, relapse prevention, self-care activities, resources, conflict management, problem-solving skills, stress management and relaxation techniques, and crisis management.

- Integrates current knowledge and research regarding psychotherapeutic educational strategies and content.

- Engages consumer alliances and advocacy groups, as appropriate, in health teaching and health promotion activities.

- Identifies community resources to assist consumers in using prevention and mental healthcare services appropriately.

- Seeks opportunities for feedback and evaluation of the effectiveness of strategies utilized.

- Provides anticipatory guidance to individuals and families to promote mental health and to prevent or reduce the risk of psychiatric disorders.

Additional Measurement Criteria for the Psychiatric-Mental Health Advanced Practice Registered Nurse

The APRN-PMH:

- Educates patients and significant others about intended effects and potential adverse effects of treatment options.

- Provides education to individuals, families, and groups to promote knowledge, understanding, and effective management of overall

Continued ▶

health maintenance, mental health problems, and psychiatric disorders.

- Uses knowledge of health beliefs, practices, evidence-based findings, and epidemiological principles, along with the social, cultural, and political issues that affect mental health in the community, to develop health promotion strategies.

- Synthesizes empirical evidence on risk behaviors, learning theories, behavioral change theories, motivational theories, epidemiology, and other related theories and frameworks when designing health information and patient education.

- Designs health information and patient education appropriate to the patient's developmental level, learning needs, readiness to learn, and cultural values and beliefs.

- Evaluates health information resources, such as the Internet, in the area of practice for accuracy, readability, and comprehensibility to help patients access quality health information.

STANDARD 5C. MILIEU THERAPY

The Psychiatric-Mental Health Registered Nurse provides, structures, and maintains a safe and therapeutic environment in collaboration with patients, families, and other healthcare clinicians.

Measurement Criteria

The Psychiatric-Mental Health Registered Nurse (RN-PMH):

- Orients the patient and family to the care environment, including the physical environment, the roles of different healthcare providers, how to be involved in the treatment and care delivery processes, schedules of events pertinent to their care and treatment, and expectations regarding behaviors.

- Orients the patient to their rights and responsibilities particular to the treatment or care environment.

- Conducts ongoing assessments of the patient in relationship to the environment to guide nursing interventions in maintaining a safe environment and patient safety.

- Selects specific activities that meet the patient's physical and mental health needs for meaningful participation in the milieu and promoting personal growth.

- Ensures that the patient is treated in the least restrictive environment necessary to maintain the safety of the patient and others.

- Informs the patient in a culturally competent manner about the need for the limits and the conditions necessary to remove the restrictions.

- Provides support and validation to patients when discussing their illness experience, and seeks to prevent complications of illness.

STANDARD 5D. PHARMACOLOGICAL, BIOLOGICAL, AND INTEGRATIVE THERAPIES

The Psychiatric-Mental Health Registered Nurse incorporates knowledge of pharmacological, biological, and complementary interventions with applied clinical skills to restore the patient's health and prevent further disability.

Measurement Criteria

The Psychiatric-Mental Health Registered Nurse (RN-PMH):

- Applies current research findings to guide nursing actions related to pharmacology, other biological therapies, and integrative therapies.

- Assesses patient's response to biological interventions based on current knowledge of pharmacological agents' intended actions, interactive effects, potential untoward effects, and therapeutic doses.

- Includes health teaching for medication management to support patients in managing their own medications and adhering to pre-scribed regimen.

- Provides health teaching about mechanism of action, intended effects, potential adverse effects of the proposed prescription, ways to cope with transitional side effects, and other treatment options, including no treatment.

- Directs interventions toward alleviating untoward effects of biological interventions.

- Communicates observations about the patient's response to biological interventions to other health clinicians.

STANDARD 5E. PRESCRIPTIVE AUTHORITY AND TREATMENT

The Psychiatric-Mental Health Advanced Practice Registered Nurse uses prescriptive authority, procedures, referrals, treatments, and therapies in accordance with state and federal laws and regulations.

Measurement Criteria

The Psychiatric-Mental Health Advanced Practice Registered Nurse (APRN-PMH):

• Conducts a thorough assessment of past medication trials, side effects, efficacy, and patient preference.

• Educates and assists the patient in selecting the appropriate use of complementary and alternative therapies.

• Provides patients with information about intended effects and potential adverse effects of proposed prescriptive therapies.

• Provides information about pharmacologic agents, costs, and alternative treatments and procedures as appropriate.

• Prescribes evidence-based treatments, therapies, and procedures considering the patient's comprehensive healthcare needs.

• Prescribes pharmacologic agents based on a current knowledge of pharmacology and physiology.

• Prescribes specific pharmacological agents and treatments based on clinical indicators, the patient's status and needs, and the results of diagnostic and laboratory tests.

• Evaluates therapeutic and potential adverse effects of pharmacological and non-pharmacological treatments.

• Evaluates pharmacological outcomes by utilizing standard symptom measurements and patient reports to determine efficacy.

STANDARD 5F. PSYCHOTHERAPY

The Psychiatric-Mental Health Advanced Practice Registered Nurse conducts individual, couples, group, and family psychotherapy using evidence-based psychotherapeutic frameworks and nurse–patient therapeutic relationships.

Measurement Criteria

The Psychiatric-Mental Health Advanced Practice Registered Nurse (APRN-PMH):

- Uses knowledge of relevant biological, psychosocial, and developmental theories, as well as best available research evidence, to select therapeutic methods based on patient needs.

- Utilizes interventions that promote mutual trust to build a therapeutic treatment alliance.

- Empowers patients to be active participants in treatment.

- Applies therapeutic communication strategies based on theories and research evidence to reduce emotional distress, facilitate cognitive and behavioral change, and foster personal growth.

- Uses awareness of own emotional reactions and behavioral responses to others to enhance the therapeutic alliance.

- Analyzes the impact of duty to report and other advocacy actions on the therapeutic alliance.

- Arranges for the provision of care in the therapist's absence.

- Applies ethical and legal principles to the treatment of patients with mental health problems and psychiatric disorders.

- Makes referrals when it is determined that the patient will benefit from a transition of care or consultation due to change in clinical condition.

- Evaluates effectiveness of interventions in relation to outcomes using standardized methods as appropriate.

- Monitors outcomes of therapy and adjusts the plan of care when indicated.

- Therapeutically concludes the nurse–patient relationship and transitions the patient to other levels of care, when appropriate.

- Manages professional boundaries in order to preserve the integrity of the therapeutic process.

STANDARD 5G. CONSULTATION

The Psychiatric-Mental Health Advanced Practice Registered Nurse provides consultation to influence the identified plan, enhance the abilities of other clinicians to provide services for patients, and effect change.

Measurement Criteria

The Psychiatric-Mental Health Advanced Practice Registered Nurse (APRN-PMH):

- Initiates consultation at the request of the consultee.

- Establishes a working alliance with the patient or consultee based on mutual respect and role responsibilities.

- Facilitates the effectiveness of a consultation by involving the stakeholders in the decision-making process.

- Synthesizes clinical data, theoretical frameworks, and evidence when providing consultation.

- Communicates consultation recommendations that influence the identified plan, facilitate understanding by involved stakeholders, enhance the work of others, and effect change.

- Clarifies that implementation of system changes or changes to the plan of care remain the consultee's responsibility.

STANDARD 6. EVALUATION
The Psychiatric-Mental Health Registered Nurse evaluates progress toward attainment of expected outcomes.

Measurement Criteria

The Psychiatric-Mental Health Registered Nurse (RN-PMH):

- Conducts a systematic, ongoing, and criterion-based evaluation of the outcomes in relation to the structures and processes prescribed by the plan and indicated timeline.

- Involves the patient, family or significant others, and other health-care clinicians in the evaluation process.

- Documents results of the evaluation.

- Evaluates the effectiveness of the planned strategies in relation to patient responses and the attainment of the expected outcomes.

- Uses ongoing assessment data to revise the diagnoses, plan, implementation, and outcomes as needed.

- Disseminates the results to the patient and others involved in the care or situation, as appropriate, in accordance with state and federal laws and regulations.

Additional Measurement Criteria for the Psychiatric-Mental Health Advanced Practice Nurse

The APRN-PMH:

- Evaluates the accuracy of the diagnosis and effectiveness of the interventions in relationship to the patient's attainment of expected outcomes.

- Synthesizes the results of the evaluation analyses to determine the impact of the plan on the affected patients, families, groups, communities, and institutions.

- Uses the results of the evaluation analyses to make or recommend process or structural changes, including policy, procedure, or protocol documentation, as appropriate.

STANDARDS OF PROFESSIONAL PERFORMANCE

STANDARD 7. QUALITY OF PRACTICE
The Psychiatric-Mental Health Registered Nurse systematically enhances the quality and effectiveness of nursing practice.

Measurement Criteria

The Psychiatric-Mental Health Registered Nurse (RN-PMH):

- Demonstrates quality by documenting the application of the nursing process in a responsible, accountable, and ethical manner.

- Uses the results of quality improvement activities to initiate changes in nursing practice and in the healthcare delivery system.

- Uses creativity and innovation in nursing practice to improve care delivery.

- Incorporates new knowledge to initiate changes in nursing practice if desired outcomes are not achieved.

- Participates in quality improvement activities. Such activities may include:

  - Identifying aspects of practice important for quality monitoring.

  - Using indicators developed to monitor quality and effectiveness of nursing practice.

  - Collecting data to monitor quality and effectiveness of nursing practice.

  - Analyzing quality data to identify opportunities for improving nursing practice.

  - Formulating recommendations to improve nursing practice or outcomes.

  - Implementing activities to enhance the quality of nursing practice.

  - Developing, implementing, and evaluating policies, procedures, and guidelines to improve the quality of practice.

Continued ▶

- Participating on interdisciplinary teams to evaluate clinical care or health services.

- Participating in efforts to minimize costs and unnecessary duplication.

- Analyzing factors related to safety, satisfaction, effectiveness, and cost–benefit options.

- Analyzing organizational systems for barriers.

- Implementing processes to remove or decrease barriers within organizational systems.

Additional Measurement Criteria for the Psychiatric-Mental Health Advanced Practice Nurse

The APRN-PMH:

- Obtains and maintains professional certification at the advanced level in psychiatric-mental health nursing.

- Designs quality improvement initiatives.

- Implements initiatives to evaluate the need for change.

- Evaluates the practice environment and quality of nursing care rendered in relation to existing evidence, identifying opportunities for the generation and use of research.

STANDARD 8. EDUCATION

The Psychiatric-Mental Health Registered Nurse attains knowledge and competency that reflect current nursing practice.

Measurement Criteria

The Psychiatric-Mental Health Registered Nurse (RN-PMH) :

- Participates in ongoing educational activities related to appropriate knowledge bases and professional issues.

- Demonstrates a commitment to lifelong learning through self-reflection and inquiry to identify learning needs.

- Seeks experiences that reflect current practice in order to maintain skills and competence in clinical practice or role performance.

- Acquires knowledge and skills appropriate to the specialty area, practice setting, role, or situation.

- Maintains professional records that provide evidence of competency and lifelong learning.

- Seeks experiences and formal and independent learning activities to maintain and develop clinical and professional skills and knowledge.

Additional Measurement Criteria for the Psychiatric-Mental Health Advanced Practice Nurse

The APRN-PMH:

- Uses current healthcare research findings and other evidence to expand clinical knowledge, enhance role performance, and increase knowledge of professional issues.

STANDARD 9: PROFESSIONAL PRACTICE EVALUATION

The Psychiatric-Mental Health Registered Nurse evaluates one's own practice in relation to the professional practice standards and guidelines, relevant statutes, rules, and regulations.

Measurement Criteria

The Psychiatric-Mental Health Registered Nurse (RN-PMH):

- Applies knowledge of current practice standards, guidelines, statutes, rules, and regulations.

- Engages in self-evaluation of practice on a regular basis, identifying areas of strength as well as areas in which professional development would be beneficial.

- Obtains informal feedback regarding practice from patients, peers, professional colleagues, and others.

- Participates in systematic peer review as appropriate.

- Takes action to achieve goals identified during the evaluation process.

- Provides rationale for practice beliefs, decisions, and actions as part of the informal and formal evaluation processes.

Additional Measurement Criteria for the Psychiatric-Mental Health Advanced Practice Registered Nurse

The APRN-PMH:

- Engages in a formal process seeking feedback regarding one's own practice from patients, peers, professional colleagues, and others.

STANDARD 10. COLLEGIALITY
The Psychiatric-Mental Health Registered Nurse interacts with and contributes to the professional development of peers and colleagues.

Measurement Criteria

The Psychiatric-Mental Health Registered Nurse (RN-PMH):

- Shares knowledge and skills with peers and colleagues as evidenced by such activities as patient care conferences or presentations at formal or informal meetings.

- Provides peers with feedback regarding their practice and role performance.

- Interacts with peers and colleagues to enhance one's own professional nursing practice and role performance.

- Maintains compassionate and caring relationships with peers and colleagues.

- Contributes to an environment that is conducive to the education of healthcare professionals.

- Contributes to a supportive and healthy work environment.

Additional Measurement Criteria for the Psychiatric-Mental Health Advanced Practice Nurse

The APRN-PMH:

- Models expert practice to interdisciplinary team members and healthcare consumers.

- Mentors other registered nurses and colleagues as appropriate.

- Participates in interdisciplinary teams that contribute to role development and advanced nursing practice and health care.

STANDARD 11: COLLABORATION

The Psychiatric-Mental Health Registered Nurse collaborates with patients, family, and others in the conduct of nursing practice.

Measurement Criteria

The Psychiatric-Mental Health Registered Nurse (RN-PMH):

- Communicates with patient, family, and healthcare providers regarding patient care and the nurse's role in the provision of that care.

- Collaborates in creating a documented plan focused on outcomes and decisions related to care and delivery of services that indicates communication with patients, families, and others.

- Partners with others to effect change and generate positive outcomes through knowledge of the patient or situation.

- Documents referrals, including provisions for continuity of care.

- Collaborates with other healthcare providers for care beyond the nurse's scope of practice.

Additional Measurement Criteria for the Psychiatric-Mental Health Advanced Practice Registered Nurse

The APRN-PMH:

- Partners with other disciplines to enhance patient care through interdisciplinary activities such as education, consultation, management, technological development, or research opportunities.

- Facilitates an interdisciplinary process with other members of the healthcare team.

- Documents plan of care communications, rationales for plan of care changes, and collaborative discussions to improve patient care.

STANDARD 12: ETHICS
The Psychiatric-Mental Health Registered Nurse integrates ethical provisions in all areas of practice.

Measurement Criteria

The Psychiatric-Mental Health Registered Nurse (RN-PMH):

- Uses *Code of Ethics for Nurses with Interpretive Statements* (ANA, 2001) to guide practice.

- Delivers care in a manner that preserves and protects patient autonomy, dignity, and rights.

- Is aware of and avoids using the power inherent in the therapeutic relationship to influence the patient in ways not related to the treatment goals.

- Maintains patient confidentiality within legal and regulatory parameters.

- Serves as a patient advocate protecting patients' rights and assisting patients in developing skills for self advocacy.

- Maintains a therapeutic and professional patient–nurse relationship with appropriate professional role boundaries.

- Demonstrates a commitment to practicing self-care, managing stress, and connecting with self and others.

- Contributes to resolving ethical issues of patients, colleagues, or systems as evidenced in such activities as participating on ethics committees.

- Reports illegal, incompetent, or impaired practices.

Additional Measurement Criteria for the Psychiatric-Mental Health Advanced Practice Nurse

The APRN-PMH:

- Informs the patient of the risks, benefits, and outcomes of health-care regimens.

- Participates in interdisciplinary teams that address ethical risks, benefits, and outcomes.

- Promotes and maintains a system and climate that is conducive to providing ethical care.

STANDARD 13: RESEARCH
The Psychiatric-Mental Health Registered Nurse integrates research findings into practice.

Measurement Criteria

The Psychiatric-Mental Health Registered Nurse (RN-PMH):

- Utilizes the best available evidence, including research findings, to guide practice decisions.
- Actively participates in research activities at various levels appropriate to the nurse's level of education and position. Such activities may include:
  - Identifying clinical problems specific to psychiatric-mental health nursing research (patient care and nursing practice).
  - Participating in data collection (surveys, pilot projects, formal studies).
  - Participating in a formal committee or program.
  - Sharing research activities and findings with peers and others.
  - Conducting research.
  - Critically analyzing and interpreting research for application to practice.
  - Using research findings in the development of policies, procedures, and standards of practice in patient care.
  - Incorporating research as a basis for learning.

Additional Measurement Criteria for the Psychiatric-Mental Health Advanced Practice Nurse

The APRN-PMH:

- Contributes to nursing knowledge by conducting, critically appraising, or synthesizing research that discovers, examines, and evaluates knowledge, theories, criteria, and creative approaches to improve healthcare practice.
- Formally disseminates research findings through activities such as presentations, publications, consultation, and journal clubs.
- Promotes a culture that consistently integrates the best available research evidence into practice.

STANDARD 14. RESOURCE UTILIZATION
The Psychiatric-Mental Health Registered Nurse considers factors related to safety, effectiveness, cost, and impact on practice in the planning and delivery of nursing services.

Measurement Criteria

The Psychiatric-Mental Health Registered Nurse (RN-PMH):

- Evaluates factors such as safety, effectiveness, availability, cost–benefit, efficiencies, and impact on practice when choosing practice options that would result in the same expected outcome.

- Assists the patient and family in identifying and securing appropriate and available services to address health-related needs.

- Assigns or delegates tasks, based on the needs and condition of the patient, potential for harm, stability of the patient's condition, complexity of the task, and predictability of the outcome.

- Assists the patient and family in becoming informed about the options, costs, risks, and benefits of treatment and care.

Additional Measurement Criteria for the Psychiatric-Mental Health Advanced Practice Nurse

The APRN-PMH:

- Utilizes organizational and community resources to formulate multidisciplinary or interdisciplinary plans of care.

- Develops innovative solutions for patient care problems that address effective resource utilization and maintenance of quality.

- Develops evaluation strategies to demonstrate quality, cost effectiveness, cost–benefit, and efficiency factors associated with nursing practice.

STANDARD 15. LEADERSHIP
The Psychiatric-Mental Health Registered Nurse provides leadership in the professional practice setting and the profession.

Measurement Criteria

The Psychiatric-Mental Health Registered Nurse (RN-PMH):

- Engages in teamwork as a team player and a team builder.

- Works to create and maintain healthy work environments in local, regional, national, or international communities.

- Displays the ability to define a clear vision with associated goals and a plan to implement and measure progress.

- Demonstrates a commitment to continuous lifelong learning for self and others.

- Teaches others to succeed by mentoring and other strategies.

- Exhibits creativity and flexibility through times of change.

- Demonstrates energy, excitement, and a passion for quality work.

- Uses mistakes by self and others as opportunities for learning so that appropriate risk-taking is encouraged.

- Inspires loyalty by valuing people as the most precious asset in an organization.

- Directs the coordination of care across settings and among caregivers, including oversight of licensed and unlicensed personnel in any assigned or delegated tasks.

- Serves in key roles in the work setting by participating on committees, councils, and administrative teams.

- Promotes advancement of the profession through participation in professional organizations.

Additional Measurement Criteria for the Psychiatric-Mental Health Advanced Practice Nurse

The APRN-PMH:

- Utilizes ethical principles to advocate for access and parity of services for mental health problems, psychiatric disorders, and addiction services.

- Influences health policy to reduce the impact of stigma on services for prevention and treatment of mental health problems and psychiatric disorders.

- Works to influence decision-making bodies to improve patient care.

- Provides direction to enhance the effectiveness of the healthcare team.

- Initiates and revises protocols or guidelines to reflect evidence-based practice, to reflect accepted changes in care management, or to address emerging problems.

- Promotes communication of information and advancement of the profession through writing, publishing, and presentations for professional or lay audiences.

- Designs innovations to effect change in practice and improve health outcomes.

REFERENCES

American Nurses Association (ANA). (2000). *Scope and standards of psychiatric-mental health nursing practice.* Washington, DC: American Nurses Publishing.

American Nurses Association (ANA). (2001). *Code of ethics for nurses with interpretive statements.* Washington, DC: American Nurses Publishing.

American Nurses Association (ANA). (2003). *Nursing's social policy statement*, 2nd ed. Washington, DC: Nursesbooks.org.

American Nurses Association (ANA). (2004). *Nursing: Scope and standards of practice.* Silver Spring, MD: Nursesbooks.org.

Anthony, W., Cohen, M., Farkas, M. & Cagne, C. (2002). *Psychiatric rehabilitation,* 2nd ed. Boston: Center for Psychiatric Rehabilitation.

Barker, P. (2001). The tidal model: Developing a person-centered approach to psychiatric-mental health nursing. *Perspectives in Psychiatric Care, 37*, 79–87.

Bigbee, H.L., & Amidi-Nouri, A. (2000). History and evolution of advanced practice nursing. In A.B. Hamric, J.A. Spross, and C.M. Hanson (Eds.), *Advanced practice: An integrative approach,* 2nd ed., pp. 3–31. Philadelphia: W.B. Saunders.

Bjorklund, P. (2003). The certified psychiatric nurse practitioner: Advanced practice psychiatric nursing reclaimed. *Archives of Psychiatric Nursing, 17*(2), 77–87.

Buckwalter, K.C., & Church, O.M. (1979). Euphemia Jane Taylor: An uncommon psychiatric nurse. *Perspectives in Psychiatric Care, XVII*, (3), 125–131.

Caplan, G., & Caplan, R.B. (1993). *Mental health consultation and collaboration*, 1st ed. San Francisco: Jossey-Bass.

Carlson-Sabelli, L., & Delaney, K.R. (2005). *Using technology to create the 21st-century practitioner*. Paper presented at the Annual Conference of the American Psychiatric Nurses Association, Nashville, Tennessee.

Chafetz, L., White, M., Collins-Bride, G., & Nickens, J. (2005). The poor general health of the severely mentally ill: Impact of schizophrenic diagnosis. *Community Mental Health Journal, 41*(2), 169–184.

Chochinov, H.M. (2001). Depression in cancer patients. *Lancet Oncology, 2,* 499–505.

Church, O.M. (1982). *That noble reform: The emergence of psychiatric nursing in the United States 1882–1963*. Dissertation. Ann Arbor: University of Michigan Dissertation Services.

Daniels, A., & Adams, N. (2004). *From Policy to Service: A Quality Vision for Behavioral Health: Using the Quality Chasm and New Freedom Commission Reports as a Framework for Change*. American College of Mental Health Administration.

deGroot, M., Anderson, R., Freedland, K.E., Clouse, R.E., & Lustman, P.J. (2001). Association of depression and diabetes complications: A meta-analysis. *Psychosomatic Medicine, 63,* 619–630.

Delaney, K.R. (2005). Evidence base for practice: Reduction of restraint and seclusion use during child and adolescent psychiatric inpatient treatment. *Journal of World-Wide Evidence*, in press.

Delaney, K.R.,Chisholm, M., Clement, J., & Merwin, E.I. (1999). Trends in psychiatric nursing education. *Archives of Psychiatric Nursing, XI*(5), 231–236.

deVries, M.W., & Wilkerson, B. (2003). Stress, work and mental health: A global perspective. *NeuroPsychiatrica, 15*(1), 44.

Draucker, C.B. (2005). Processes of mental health service use by adolescents with depression. *Journal of Nursing Scholarship, 37,* 155–162.

Duffy, F.F., West, J.C., Kohut, J.J., Pion, G.M., Wicherski, M.M., Bateman,

N., et al. (2004). Mental health practitioners and trainees. In R.W. Mandersheid & M. J. Henderson (Eds.), *Mental Health United States, 2002*, pp. 327–368. Rockville, MD: SAMHSA, DHHS Pub. No. (SMA) 3938.

Escobar-Chaves, S.L., Tortolero, S.R., Markham, C.M., Low, B.J., Eitel, P., & Thickstun, P. (2005). Impact of the media on adolescent sexual attitudes and behaviors. *Pediatrics, 116*(1), 303–326.

Fawzy, F.I., Fawzy, N.W., Hyun, C.S., Elashoff, R., Guthrie, D., Fahey, J.L., et al. (1993). Malignant melanoma. Effects of an early structured psychiatric intervention, coping, and affective state on recurrence and survival 6 years later. *Archives of General Psychiatry, 50,* 681–689.

Forchuck, C., Martin, M.L., Chan, Y.L., & Jensen, E. (2005). Therapeutic relationships: From psychiatric hospital to community. *Journal of Psychiatric-Mental Health Nursing, 12*(5), 556–564.

Haber, J., & Billings, C.V. (1995). Primary mental health care: A vision for the future of psychiatric-mental health nursing. *Journal of the American Psychiatric Nurses Association, 1,* 154–163.

Hanrahan, N.P., & Sullivan-Marx, E. M. (2005). Practice patterns and potential solutions to the shortage of providers of older adult mental health services. *Policy, Politics and Nursing Practice, 6*(3), 1–10.

Hauenstein, E.J. (1997). A nursing practice paradigm for depressed rural women: The Women's Affective Illness Treatment Program. *Archives of Psychiatric Nursing, 11,* 37–45.

Institute of Medicine (IOM). (2005). *Improving the quality of health care for mental and substance-use conditions: Quality chasm series.* Retrieved April, 2007, from http://www.iom.edu/cms/3809/19405/30836.aspx.

Johnson, M.E., & Delaney, K.R. (2006). Keeping the unit safe: A grounded theory study. *Journal of the American Psychiatric Nurses Association 12,* 13–21.

Kaas, M.J., & Markley, J.M. (1998). A national perspective on prescriptive authority for advanced practice nurses. *Journal of the American Psychiatric Nurses Association, 4,* 190–198.

Kessler, R.C., Demler, O., Frank, R.G., Olfson, M., Pincus, H.A., Walters, E.E., et al.(2005).Prevalence and treatment of mental disorders 1900–2003. *New England Journal of Medicine, 352*(24), 2515–2523.

Kestenbaum, C. (2000). How shall we treat children in the 21st Century? *Journal of the American Academy of Child and Adolescent Psychiatry, 39* (1), 1–10.

Koike, A.K., Unutzer, J., & Wells, K.B. (2002). Improving care for depression in patients with co-morbid medical illness. *American Journal of Psychiatry, 159*(10), 1738–1745.

Kuijpers, P., Van Straten, A., & Smit, F. (2005). Preventing the incidence of new cases of mental disorders. *Journal of Nervous and Mental Disease, 193*, 119–125.

Manderscheid, R.W., Atay, J.E., Male, A., Blacklow, B., Forest, C., Ingram, L., Maedke, J., et al. (2004). Highlights of organized mental health services in 2000 and major national and state trends. In R.W. Mandersheid & M. J. Henderson (Eds.), *Mental Health United States, 2002*. DHHS Pub. No. (SMA) 3938. Retrieved February 16, 2007, from http://www.mentalhealth.samhsa.gov/publications/allpubs/SMA04-3938/default.asp.

Martin, A., & Leslie, D. (2003). Psychiatric inpatient, outpatient, and medication utilization and costs among privately insured youths, 1997–2000. *American Journal of Psychiatry, 160*, 757–764.

McGrew, J.H., & Bond, G.R. (1995). Critical ingredients of assertive community treatment: Judgments of the experts. *Journal of Mental Health Administration, 22*, 113–125.

McGuiness, T.M. & Noonan, P. (2004). Top ten reasons to take your graduate program in psychiatric nursing online. *Journal of Psychosocial Nursing and Mental Health Services, 42*(12), 33–38.

Messer, S. B. (2006). Patient values and preferences. In J. C. Norcross, L. E. Beutler, & R. L. Levant (Eds.), *Evidence-based practice in mental health: Debate and dialogue on fundamental questions*, pp. 31–40. Washington, DC: American Psychology Press.

Mrazek, P.J., & Hagerty, R.J. (1994). *Reducing risks for mental disorders*. Washington, DC: National Academy Press.

National Association of Psychiatric Health Systems. (2003). *Challenges facing behavioral health care: The pressures on essential behavioral healthcare services*. Retrieved February 16, 2007 from http://www.naphs.org/news/whitepaper4031.pdf.

National Panel for Psychiatric-Mental Health NP Competencies. (2003). *Psychiatric-mental health nurse practitioner competencies*. Washington, DC: National Organization of Nurse Practitioner Faculties. Retrieved February 16, 2007 from http://www.nonpf.com/finalcomps03.pdf.

New Freedom Commission on Mental Health. (2003). *Achieving the promise: Transforming mental health care in America. Final report*. DHHS Pub. No. SMA-03-3832. Rockville, MD: Department of Health and Human Services. http://www.mentalhealthcommission.gov/reports/FinalReport/toc.html

Norcross, J.C., Beutler, L.E., & Levant, R.L. (2005). Prologue. In J. C. Norcross, L. E., Beutler, L. E., & R. L. Levant (Eds.), *Evidence-based practice in mental health: Debate and dialogue on fundamental questions,* pp. 3–12. Washington, DC: American Psychology Press.

O'Brien, A.J. (2001). The therapeutic relationship: Historical development and contemporary significance. *Journal of Psychiatric and Mental Health Nursing, 8,* 129–137.

Olfson M., Marcus, S.C., Druss, B., et al. (2002). National trends in the outpatient treatment of depression. *Journal of the American Medical Association 287*(2):203–209.

Persky, T. (1998). Overlooked and underserved: Elders in need of mental health care. *Journal of the California Alliance for the Mentally Ill, 9,* 7–9.

Pestka, E. (2003) Genetic core competencies: Exploring the implications for psychiatric nursing. *Journal of the American Psychiatric Nurses Association, 9,* 1–8.

Phillips, S.D., Burns, B.J., Edgar, E.R., Mueser, K.T., Linkins, K.W., Rosenheck, R.A., et al. (2001). Moving assertive community treatment into standard practice. *Psychiatric Services, 52*, 771–779.

Pottick, K.J., Warner, L.A., Isaacs, M., Henderson, M.J., Milazzo-Sayre, L., & Manderscheid, R.W. (2002). Children and adolescents admitted to specialty mental health programs in the United States, 1986 and 1997. In R.W. Mandersheid & M. J. Henderson (Eds.), *Mental health United States, 2002.* Rockville, MD: SAMHSA, DHHS Pub. No. (SMA) 3938.

Raingruber, B. (1999). Recognizing, understanding and responding to familiar responses: The importance of relationship history for therapeutic effectiveness. *Perspectives in Psychiatric Care, 35*, 5–17.

Raingruber, B. (2003). Nurture: The fundamental significance of relationship as a paradigm for mental health nursing. *Perspectives in Psychiatric Care, 39*, 104–112, 132–135.

Rapp, C.A. (1998). The active ingredients of effective case management: A research synthesis. *Community Mental Health Journal, 43*, 363–380.

Sackett, D.L. (2000). *Evidence-based medicine: How to practice and teach EBM,* 2nd ed. New York: Churchville Livingstone.

Salyers, M.P., & Macy, V.R. (2005). Recovery-oriented evidence-based practices: A commentary. *Community Mental Health Journal, 41*, 101–103.

Sapolsky, R.M. (2003). Gene therapy for psychiatric disorders. *American Journal of Psychiatry, 160*, 208–220.

Sephton, S.E., Sapolsky, R.M., Kraemer, H.C., & Spiegel, D. (2000). Diurnal cortisol rhythm as a predictor of breast cancer survival. *Journal of the National Cancer Institute, 92,* 994–1000.

Society for Education and Research in Psychiatric Nursing (SERPN). (2005). International Society of Psychiatric-Mental Health Nurses (ISPN).

Spear, S.J. (2005). Fixing health care from the inside, today. *Harvard Business Review*, September, 78–91.

Stark, D.P. & House, A. (2000). Anxiety in cancer patients. *British Journal of Cancer, 83,* 1261–1267.

Stuart, G.W., Tondora, J., & Hoge, M.A. (2004). Evidence-based teaching practice: Implications for behavioral health. *Administration & Policy in Mental Health, 32* (2), 107–130.

Substance Abuse and Mental Health Services Administration (SAMHSA). (2005). *Transforming mental health care in America. The Federal Action Agenda: First Steps.* DHHS Pub. No. SMA-05-4060. Rockville, MD: SAMHSA.

Taylor, C.M. (1999). Introduction to psychiatric-mental health nursing. In P. O'Brien, W.Z. Kennedy, & K.A. Ballard (Eds.), *Psychiatric nursing: An integration of theory and practice,* pp. 3–19. New York: McGraw-Hill.

U.S. Census Bureau. (2004). *Census Bureau projects tripling of Hispanic and Asian populations in 50 years; Non-Hispanic whites may drop to half of total population.* Retrieved February 16, 2007 from http://www.census.gov/Press-Release/www/releases/archives/population/001720.html.

U.S. Department of Health and Human Services (U.S. DHHS). (2001). *Mental Health: Culture, Race and Ethnicity—A Supplement to Mental Health: A Report of the Surgeon General.* Rockville, MD: U.S. Department of Health and Human Services, Substance Abuse and Mental Health Services Administration, Center for Mental Health Services.

Wheeler, K., & Haber, J. (2004). Development of psychiatric-mental health nurse practitioner competencies: Opportunities for the 21st century. *Journal of the American Psychiatric Nurses Association, 10*(3), 129–138.

Whyte, E.M., & Mulsant, B.H. (2002). Post-stroke depression: Epidemiology, pathophysiology, and biological treatment. *Biological Psychiatry, 52*(3), 253–264.

World Health Organization (WHO). (2001). *The world health report 2001—Mental health: New understanding, new hope.* Geneva: WHO.

World Health Organization (WHO). (2002). *Reducing risks, promoting healthy life.* Geneva: WHO.

GLOSSARY

Assessment. A systematic, dynamic process by which the registered nurse, through interaction with the patient, family, groups, communities, populations, and healthcare providers, collects and analyzes data. Assessment may include the following dimensions: physical, psychological, socio-cultural, spiritual, cognitive, functional abilities, developmental, economic, and lifestyle.

Caregiver. A person who provides direct care for another, such as a child, dependent adult, the disabled, or the chronically ill.

Clinical supervision. The process in which one mental health professional seeks assistance from another to discuss therapeutic issues or to identify or clarify a concern or problem and to consider alternatives for problem resolution.

Continuity of care. An interdisciplinary process that includes patients, families, and significant others in the development of a coordinated plan of care. This process facilitates the patient's transition between settings and healthcare providers, based on changing needs and available resources.

Counseling. A specific, time-limited interaction of a nurse with a patient, family, or group experiencing immediate or ongoing difficulties related to their health or well-being. The difficulty is investigated using a problem-solving approach for the purpose of understanding the experience and integrating it with other life experiences.

Crisis intervention. A short-term therapeutic process that focuses on the rapid resolution of an immediate crisis or emergency using available personnel, family, and/or environmental resources.

Criteria. Relevant, measurable indicators of the standards of practice and professional performance.

Diagnosis. A clinical judgment about the patient's response to actual or potential health conditions or needs. The diagnosis provides the basis for determination of a plan to achieve expected outcomes. Registered nurses utilize nursing or medical diagnoses depending upon educational and clinical preparation and legal authority.

Environment. The atmosphere, milieu, or conditions in which an individual lives, works, or plays.

Evaluation. The process of determining the progress toward attainment of expected outcomes, including the effectiveness of care, when addressing one's practice.

Evidence-based practice. A process founded on the collection, interpretation, and integration of valid, important, and applicable patient-reported, clinician-observed, and research-derived evidence. The best available evidence, moderated by patient circumstances and preferences, is applied to improve the quality of clinical judgments.

Family. Family of origin or significant others as identified by the patient.

Guidelines. Systematically developed statements that describe recommended actions based on available scientific evidence and expert opinion. Clinical guidelines describe a process of patient care management that has the potential of improving the quality of clinical and consumer decision-making.

Health. An experience that is often expressed in terms of wellness and illness, and may occur in the presence or absence of disease or injury.

Healthcare providers. Individuals with special expertise who provide healthcare services or assistance to patients. They may include nurses, physicians, psychologists, social workers, nutritionist/dietitians, and various therapists.

Holistic. Based on an understanding that the parts of a patient are intimately interconnected and physical, mental, social, and spiritual factors need to be included in any interventions.

Illness. The subjective experience of discomfort.

Implementation. Activities such as teaching, monitoring, providing, counseling, delegating, and coordinating.

Information. Data that are interpreted, experienced, or structured.

Interdisciplinary. Reliant on the overlapping skills and knowledge of each team member and discipline, resulting in synergistic effects where outcomes are enhanced and more comprehensive than the simple aggregation of the team members' individual efforts.

Interventions. Nursing activities that promote and foster health, assess dysfunction, assist patients to regain or improve their coping, abilities, and prevent further disabilities.

Knowledge. Information that is synthesized so that relationships are identified and formalized.

Mental health. Emotional and psychological wellness; the capacity to interact with others, deal with ordinary stress, and perceive one's surroundings realistically.

Mental illness/mental disorder. A disturbance in thoughts or mood that causes maladaptive behavior, inability to cope with normal stresses, and/or impaired functioning. Etiology may include genetic, physical, chemical, biological, psychological, or sociocultural factors. *Mental illness* covers all mental disorders.

Multidisciplinary. Reliant on each team member or discipline contributing discipline-specific skills.

Nursing process. A nursing methodology based on critical thinking. The steps consist of assessment, diagnosis, outcomes identification, planning, implementation, and evaluation.

Outcomes. The patient's goal, or the result of interventions, that includes the degree of wellness and the continued need for care, medication, support, counseling, education.

Patient. Recipient of nursing practice. The term *patient* is used to provide consistency and brevity, bearing in mind that other terms such as *client, individual, resident, family, group, community,* or *population* may be better choices in some instances. When the patient is an individual, the focus is on the health state, problems, or needs of the individual. When the patient is a family or group, the focus is on the health state of the unit as a whole or the reciprocal effects of the individual's health state on the other members of the unit. When the patient is a community or population, the focus is on personal and environmental health and the health risks of the community or population.

Plan. A comprehensive outline of the steps that need to be completed to attain expected outcomes.

Psychiatric disorder. Any condition of the brain that adversely affects the patient's cognition, emotions, or behavior.

Psychiatric-Mental Health Advanced Practice Registered Nurse (APRN-PMH). A licensed registered nurse who is educationally prepared at the master's or doctorate level in the specialty of psychiatric-mental health nursing, holds ANCC advanced practice specialty certification, and demonstrates a depth and breadth of knowledge and a greater synthesis of data, increased complexity of skills and interventions, and significant role autonomy than the RN. APRN-PMH practice focuses on applying competencies, knowledge, and experience to individuals, families, or groups with complex psychiatric-mental health problems, promoting mental health in society, and collaborating with and doing referrals to other health professionals as dictated by either the patient's need or the APRN-PMH's practice focus.

Psychotherapy. A formally structured, contractual relationship between the therapist and patient(s) for the purpose of effecting change in the patient system. Approaches include all generally accepted and respected methods of therapy, including individual therapy (play and other expressive therapies, insight therapy, behavioral therapy, cognitive therapy, and brief goal- or solution-oriented therapy), group therapy, couple/marital therapy, and family therapy.

Quality of care. The degree to which health services for patients, families, groups, communities, or populations increase the likelihood of desired outcomes and are consistent with current professional knowledge.

Recovery. A way of living a satisfying, hopeful, and contributing life even with the limitations caused by illness. Recovery involves the development of new meaning and purpose in one's life as one grows beyond the catastrophic events of mental illness.

Standard. An authoritative statement defined and promoted by the profession, by which the quality of practice, service, or education can be evaluated.

Therapeutic process. The use of the nurse–patient relationship and the nursing process to promote and maintain a patient's adaptive coping responses

APPENDIX A.
SCOPE AND STANDARDS OF PSYCHIATRIC-MENTAL HEALTH NURSING PRACTICE (2000)

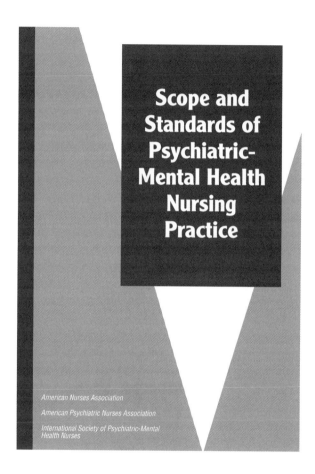

Scope and
Standards of
Psychiatric-
Mental Health
Nursing
Practice

American Nurses Association
American Psychiatric Nurses Association
International Society of Psychiatric-Mental
Health Nurses

SCOPE and STANDARDS
of
Psychiatric-Mental Health
Nursing Practice

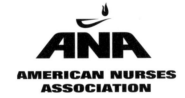

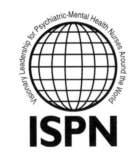

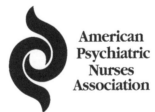

Washington, D.C.

Library of Congress Cataloging-in-Publication Data

American Nurses' Association
    Scope and standards of psychiatric-mental health nursing practice /
American Nurses Association, American Psychiatric Nurses Association,
International Society of Psychiatric-Mental Health Nurses.
        p. ; cm.
    Includes bibliographical references.
    ISBN 1-55810-153-5
        1. Psychiatric nursing—United States. 2. Psychiatric nursing—
Standards—United States. I. American Psychiatric Nurses Association.
II. International Society of Psychiatric-Mental Health Nurses. III. Title.
        [DNLM: 1. Psychiatric Nursing—standards—United States.
    2. Nursing Care—standards—United States. WY 160 A5127s 2000]
RC440 .A565 2000
610.73'68'021873—dc21   00-055880

Published by
American Nurses Publishing
600 Maryland Avenue, SW
Suite 100 West
Washington, DC 20024-2571

ISBN 1-55810-153-5

PMH-20   5M   09/00

ACKNOWLEDGMENTS

The American Nurses Association gratefully acknowledges all the valuable assistance, comments, and recommendations given by various individuals and groups across the country who have collaborated throughout this revision process.

Workgroup to Review and Revise the Statement on *Psychiatric-Mental Health Nursing Practice and Standards of Psychiatric-Mental Health Clinical Nursing Practice*

Grayce Sills, PhD, RN, FAAN, Chairperson
American Nurses Association

Karen A. Ballard, MA, RN
ANA Standards and Guidelines Committee

Carolyn V. Billings, MSN, RN,CS
American Psychiatric Nurses Association

Peggy E. Dulaney, MSN, RN,CS
International Society of Psychiatric-Mental Health Nurses

Jane B. Neese, PhD, RN,CS
ISPN, Society for Education and Research
in Psychiatric-Mental Health Nursing Division

Peggy Plunkett, MSN, ARNP, CS
ISPN, International Society for
Psychiatric Consultation Liaison Nurses Division

Kathleen Scharer, PhD, RN,CS, FAAN
ISPN, Association of Child and
Adolescent Psychiatric Nurses Division

Carole A. Shea, PhD, RN, FAAN
American Psychiatric Nurses Association

Staff, ANA Department of Nursing Practice

Sally M. Raphel, MS, RN,CS, Director
Carol J. Bickford, PhD, RN,C, Senior Policy Fellow
Winifred Carson, JD, Nursing Practice Counsel
Yvonne Humes, BBA, Senior Administrative Assistant

CONTENTS

Acknowledgments 72

Preface 76

Introduction 77
   Contemporary Issues and Trends 77

Scope of Practice for Psychiatric-Mental Health Nursing 86
   Psychiatric-Mental Health Nursing Clinical
      Practice Activities 88
   Levels of Psychiatric-Mental Health Clinical
      Nursing Practice 89
      Basic Level 89
      Basic Level Practice 89
      Advanced Level Psychiatric-Mental Health
         Nursing Practice 93
   Psychiatric-Mental Health Nursing
      Clinical Practice Settings 98
      Community-based Care 98
      Intermediate- and Long-term Care 99
      Telehealth 100
      Self-employment 100
   Subspecialization 101
   Advocacy and Social Responsibility 101
      Advocacy 101
      Expanded Advocacy Activities .101
      Social Responsibility 102
   Psychiatric-Mental Health Nursing Ethics 102

Standards of Care 104
   Standard I. Assessment 104
   Standard II. Diagnosis 106
   Standard III. Outcome Identification 107
   Standard IV. Planning 108
   Standard V. Implementation 109
      Standard Va. Counseling 110

Standard Vb. Milieu Therapy 110
Standard Vc. Promotion of Self-Care Activities 111
Standard Vd. Psychobiological Interventions 112
Standard Ve. Health Teaching 112
Standard Vf. Case Management 113
Standard Vg. Health Promotion and
    Health Maintenance 113
Advanced Practice Interventions Vh–Vj 114
    Standard Vh. Psychotherapy 114
    Standard Vi. Prescriptive Authority and
        Treatment 115
    Standard Vj. Consultation 116
Standard VI. Evaluation 116

Standards of Professional Performance **118**
Standard I. Quality of Care 118
Standard II. Performance Appraisal 119
Standard III. Education 120
Standard IV. Collegiality 121
Standard V. Ethics 122
Standard VI. Collaboration 123
Standard VII. Research 124
Standard VIII. Resource Utilization 125

Glossary **127**

References **133**

PREFACE

The Congress on Nursing Practice and Economics has oversight responsibility to ensure currency and relevance of the published scopes and standards and has mandated a five year review of all these documents. A workgroup convened in May 1999 to review and revise, if necessary, the *Statement of Psychiatric-Mental Health Clinical Nursing Practice and the Standards of Psychiatric-Mental Health Clinical Nursing Practice* published in 1994. The current revision process, coordinated and chaired by the American Nurses Association (ANA), was a joint effort with the American Psychiatric Nurses Association and the International Society of Psychiatric-Mental Health Nurses, which now includes the divisions of the Association of Child and Adolescent Psychiatric Nurses, the Society for Education and Research in Psychiatric-Mental Health Nursing, and the International Society of Psychiatric Consultation Liaison Nurses. Each of the organizations appointed representatives, thereby assuring a depth and breadth of input from a variety of psychiatric-mental health nursing perspectives.

The field review process incorporated the innovation of posting the draft for public comment at http://www.nursingworld.org, supplementing the traditional distribution of draft paper documents to nursing specialty organizations, ANA constituent member associations, and other selected experts. Respondents included individual clinicians, groups of clinicians, undergraduate and graduate students, individual faculty members, faculty groups, faculty-student groups, and state nurses associations forwarding individual or aggregated responses from their members. After reviewing the very thoughtful responses of over 150 nurses, the workgroup members carefully integrated those recommendations into the document, thereby clarifying and strengthening the scope statement and standards of practice to truly reflect the specialty of psychiatric-mental health nursing.

INTRODUCTION

The nursing profession, by developing and articulating the scope and standards of professional nursing practice, defines its boundaries, informs society about the parameters of nursing practice, and guides states in the development of rules and regulations determining nursing practice. However, because each state creates its own laws governing nursing, the designated limits, functions, and titles for nurses, especially those in advanced practice, may vary significantly from state to state.

As always, in the case of professional practice accountability, nurses must ensure that the practice of nursing remains within their state nurse practice act, professional code of ethics, and professional practice standards. Individual nurses must ensure that their practice remains within these boundaries and within the limits of their own personal competency.

Nursing practice is also differentiated according to the nurse's educational preparation and level of practice, and is further circumscribed by the role of the nurse and the work practice setting. In addition, the nurse can focus on clinical, administrative, educative, and research responsibilities. This document specifically addresses the clinical role, clinical scope, and clinical standards of practice in the specialty area of psychiatric-mental health nursing.

Contemporary Issues and Trends

Unprecedented changes in health care practice and funding have had profound effects on psychiatric and behavioral health care, and the role of the psychiatric-mental health nurse (Shea 1999; Stuart 1997). In the 1990s, health care became a legislative priority. Politicians and policy makers undertook a vigorous national debate about necessary reforms in response to the escalating costs of health care and the increasing uninsured population. The Clinton Administration health care reform plan, although promising, ultimately failed to garner support from Congress and the public because of political factors and the complexity, scope, and projected cost of the reform plan. Yet, important consequences evolved from this initiative:

- Health care was propelled to the top of the national agenda.

- The focus shifted to primary health care delivery.

- The emphasis on health promotion and disease prevention increased.

- The needs of medically underserved and vulnerable populations were acknowledged.

- Models of managed care were developed.

- Cost containment, productivity, accountability, patient outcomes, and quality management became the operating principles for health care delivery systems.

Of these, the most notable was the advent of managed care and managed behavioral health care models (*1997 Behavioral Managed Care Sourcebook* 1996). Many of the products of managed care have become standards of the health care industry, such as practice guidelines, care paths, "report cards," consumer-friendly health education materials, extended office hours, telephone triage, and telehealth services. Despite these advances, some of the managed care models employed short-sighted, ill-conceived measures in their early attempts to control costs and increase efficiencies (Mohr 1998). Some examples were cutting professional staff, rigidly enforcing treatment protocols, and declining to provide prescribed medications and services. While proposing to manage care, in reality these models often seemed to do little more than manage cost. But with pressure from health care consumers for better health care, and legislative actions to curb detrimental operational practices, there seems to be a positive trend toward more emphasis on quality of care, as well as cost containment (Valentine 1999).

As the country began to consider a health care system that would provide primary health care services and increased access to underserved populations, it became clear that it would be necessary to enlarge the pool of health care clinicians, particularly primary health care professionals. The shift to primary health care called for more advanced, community-based clinicians, not necessarily more physicians, who were prepared to deliver primary health care services in community settings and underserved areas. Government programs, private foundations, academic institutions, and health centers partnered to develop new models to educate health professionals and deliver competency-based practice. For example, these programs were sponsored by the Bureau of Health Professions, the Centers for Disease Control and Prevention, the Pew Health Professions Commission, the Robert Wood Johnson Foundation, and the W. K. Kellogg Foundation.

During this time, nursing organizations were active participants in the national debate on health care reform and the development of new partnerships. The ANA and other professional nursing organizations established an agenda for health care, with nurses and nursing as essential ingredients to enhance access, cost-effectiveness and quality care (ANA 1991; Krauss 1993). The ANA promoted the concept of the advanced practice registered nurse (APRN) as an inclusive term for clinical nurse specialists, nurse practitioners, nurse midwives, and certified nurse anesthetists (ANA 1995). Functioning in expanded roles with increased responsibility such as prescriptive authority (Kaas and Martley 1998), APRNs greatly increased the pool of well-qualified primary care clinicians. In addition to serving as advanced practice clinicians, APRNs also made major contributions in many roles (Campbell, Musil, and Zauszniewski 1998) such as

- Clinical care manager

- Triage nurse

- Utilization reviewer

- Patient/family educator

- Case manager

- Risk manager

- Chief quality officer

- Marketing and development specialist

- Corporate manager and executive

The ANA's use of "APRN" as an umbrella term for all advanced practice nurses was a successful political strategy to educate regulators and legislators about society's need for the training and services of APRNs. However, among psychiatric-mental health nurses, it contributed to a controversy about the roles and functions of clinical nurse specialists (CNS) versus nurse practitioners (NP) (McCabe and Grover 1999). What was different about the roles? What was equivalent about the functions? Were the clinical nurse specialist and nurse practitioner roles separate and distinct, or blended (Pasacreta et al. 1999)? This document takes the position that there is a blended role (Williams et al. 1998) within one scope of practice for the psychiatric-mental health clinical nurse specialist and psychiatric-mental health nurse practitioner. The roles and functions of the APRN in psychiatric-mental health nursing are described further in the Scope of Practice section of this document.

Changes in the health care environment have had a great impact—some positive, some negative—on the way mental health services are delivered and funded. The main issues are the

- Predominance of managed behavioral health care.
- Impact of the Federal Balanced Budget Act of 1997 (PL 105-33).
- Changes in reimbursement for services.
- Needs of vulnerable populations.
- Influence of consumer and family advocates.
- Parity in insurance benefits for treatment of mental illness.
- Rapid development of genetics and scientific advances.
- Importance of global projections of mental illness.
- Significance of the publication of *Mental Health: A Report of the Surgeon General* (U.S. Department of Health and Human Services 1999).

Managed behavioral health care is the form of mental health services that dominates the treatment of mental illness (Pelletier and Beaudin 1999). Some institutions and agencies still provide mental health services within their organization (known as "carve-in" services). More frequently, mental health services are "carved-out"; that is the insurer contracts with a separate provider for mental health services, one outside the organization that provides general health care for its insured customers. The carve-out model allows for specialized mental health care only, which may disadvantage patients who also need physical care. At best, their care is fragmented. Many mental health services formerly delivered in the public sector have been contracted to the private (for-profit) sector, raising concerns about accessibility, accountability, and conflicts of interest. Furthermore, with the closing of many state mental hospitals and the deep cuts in funding to community mental health agencies, there is real concern that patients and families will not receive even a minimal level of mental health care (Mohr 1998).

Reimbursement mechanisms and productivity quotas have also radically altered the therapies used to treat mental illness (Lindeke and Chesny 1999) and limited the ability to offer preventive services. With the emphasis on evidence-based practice, mandated limits on the number of visits, and strict formularies for the prescription of psychopharmacological medications, the practice of the mental health clinician has become more standardized, potentially threatening individualized plans of care (*1997 Behavioral Managed Care Sourcebook* 1996). Short-term, time-limited, and cognitive-behavioral therapies are often the treatments of choice, and conventional medications are sometimes favored over the atypical or latest generation of medication (Dee, Servellen, and Brecht 1998). In many cases this may be very appropriate treatment, but clinicians must struggle with burdensome bureaucratic oversight and lack of flexibility and autonomy in their practice (Wurzbach 1998).

The impact of the Federal Balanced Budget Act of 1997 (Public Law 105-33) and the sweeping reform of the public welfare system has had serious consequences for health services. These laws have led to further restriction of mental health services, especially for the severely and persistently mentally ill. Programs such as Medicare, Medicaid, and disability benefits are being decreased or in some cases phased out. Those with mental illness and developmental disabilities, vulnerable populations with few resources and few social supports, are particularly hard hit by these changes (Ahmed and Maurana 1999; Collins, 1998). Without sufficient services, there will be an increase in homelessness, substance abuse, incarceration, chronic physical illness, and worsening of the individual's psychiatric condition and prognosis for change. Some other vulnerable populations that are adversely affected by the budgeted decrease in services include children and adolescents, particularly in out-of-home placements; elderly, especially home-bound elders; persons with physical disabilities; immigrants; migrant workers; residents in urban and rural underserved areas, and incarcerated persons (Farnum et al. 1999; Flaskerud and Wuerker 1999; Goldkuhle 1999; Mrazek and Haggerty 1994; U.S. Department of Health and Human Services, U.S. Public Health Service 1999; Wallace et al. 1999). The mental health and well-being of these vulnerable populations are also of concern to psychiatric nurses.

Consumer and family member advocates are major societal forces in creating pressure for change in mental health care delivery. Both groups, family members and consumers, have had serious concerns about the openness and responsiveness of clinicians and systems to their needs for information and participation in treatment decision making. The National Alliance for the Mentally Ill (NAMII), the Federation of Families, and other consumer groups have been forceful advocates for ethical care, patients' rights bills, development of more effective treatments, and greater choice of clinicians and systems of care (Wysoker 1999).

Consumer and family advocates have been some of the prime movers with respect to insurance benefits for the treatment of mental illness (Wysoker 1999). Working together with psychiatric nurses, nursing organizations, and others, the advocates helped to shape policy and legislation at the national level that addresses the need for closer parity in benefits; that is, insurance coverage of similar value, between mental health and physical health. The national plan has been augmented by legislation in many states. There is better coverage for mental illness than in the past, and in some cases, there is now coverage where none existed. However, full parity has not been achieved.

Mental health care delivery has expanded to a wide variety of sites in the community and social institutions, such as homes, schools, churches, civic centers, senior housing, work settings, courtrooms, and prisons (Rosedale 1999; Thomas, Brandt, and O'Connor 1999). Mental health treatment is also evolving a variety of approaches that consider the holistic nature of persons and systems (Laffrey and Kulbok 1999). Research supports the use of some tested complementary therapies, and some insurance companies will cover these therapies. Therefore, comprehensive care includes the use of complementary therapies, collaboration with nontraditional clinicians, and partnerships with diverse and relevant community and institutional groups (Ahmed and Maurana 1999). All of this requires that the nurse maintain clinical and cultural competence and collaborative skills through continuing education and other forms of learning (Boutain and Olivares 1999).

A continuing trend has been the expansion of knowledge and understanding of mental illness and treatment. Genetic and scientific advances have received increased attention. The scientific evidence strongly supports the biological, and genetic, as well as psychosocial explanations for the complex phenomena of psychiatric conditions (Cohen 2000). The Human Genome Project (*Understanding Our Genetic Inheritance: The U.S. Human Genome Project, The First Five Years: Fiscal Years 1991–1995,* 1990) will continue to generate findings that link genetic endowment with susceptibility to mental conditions. The counseling needs associated with genetic testing and ethical decision making indicate that psychiatric nurses can play an important role in helping patients to make informed choices about genetic testing and treatments (Donaldson 1997).

The expansion of knowledge has been limitless and continues to yield new and better methods of diagnosis and treatment for mental disorders and substance abuse (Shea et al. 1999). There are more effective psychotherapies, biologically based treatments, psychopharmacology, and complementary therapies. The development of practice guidelines, emphasis on patient outcomes, and accountability for evidence-based practice call for a clinician who is steeped in the latest research, engages in best practices, and uses the consultative role for positive patient outcomes (Smith 1999). These conditions of modern practice call for the services of psychiatric nurses.

Together with science, technology has revolutionized the way nurses and other clinicians practice mental health care (ANA 1999ab). Science and technology influence how nurses collect and analyze data, form diagnoses, plan care, identify outcomes, intervene in illness and disability, and evaluate treatment approaches and outcomes (ANA 1999a; Verhey 1999). Communication technology, such as the Internet and telehealth services, gives greater access to health care information and treatment. This open access also poses increased concerns about confidentiality and other ethical dilemmas. These ethical concerns will continue to surface as technology becomes even more woven into every aspect of work and daily life (Verhey 1999). As communication experts, psychiatric nurses are prepared to join the discussion about how society will contend with ethical issues pertaining to truly informed consent, advance directives, and rights to privacy (Sellin 1999; Wysoker, 1999). Psychiatric nurses are the human bridge between technology and the patient.

Global projections of mental illness have come to the attention of many. Demographers have predicted a worldwide increase in the aging of populations. A sizeable increase in the elder component of society will also increase the incidence of chronic illnesses and disability, such as Alzheimer's disease, in the population. The World Health Organization (WHO) (Murray and Lopez 1996) has listed unipolar depression, alcohol use, bipolar disorder, schizophrenia, and obsessive-compulsive disorder among the ten leading causes of disability worldwide. Violence and self-inflicted injuries are also ranked high among the major disabilities that will afflict global society in 2020. In all, psychiatric illnesses are projected to account for 11 to 15 percent of the global disease burden in the next century. In addition, people with severe and persistent mental illness frequently have associated substance abuse problems, especially alcoholism, as well as physical health problems that require treatment. These data suggest the growing need for more mental health services and more psychiatric clinicians.

When the effects of frequent global travel, migration and immigration patterns, ethnic conflicts, and international war are considered, it becomes clear that cultural diversity is also a significant factor in determining the provision of appropriate health care at home and abroad (Carnevale 1999). Cultural diversity within the United States continues to increase as the balance shifts toward a majority of people of color by mid-century. Language, cultural heritage, ethnic customs, and traditions have a tremendous impact on health beliefs and practices, the manifestations of psychiatric and physical illnesses, and responses to treatment and therapies. Therefore, increasing cultural competence within the nursing workforce and recruiting ethnically and racially diverse women and men into nursing will remain an important priority during the next decade (Pratt 1999).

The Surgeon General's mental health report (U.S. Department of Health and Human Services, U.S. Public Health Services 1999) is a marker event, the first Surgeon's Report to be focused on public health issues in mental health. The report specifically addresses suicide as a serious public health problem, especially for adolescents and the elderly. Suicide is the ninth leading cause of mortality in the United States. About eighty-five people commit suicide each day, with firearms causing 59 percent of the deaths (U.S. Department of Health and Human Services, U.S. Public Health Service 1999). The Surgeon General's report urges a public health approach as the national strategy to reduce suicidal behaviors and prevent premature deaths. Recommendations have implications for public awareness, education, risk assessment, prevention, intervention, training programs, and research. From the mental health perspective, this report brings to the public's attention the need to abolish the stigma of mental illness and the hope that effective treatment can give. Psychiatric nurses, as front-line care givers in community settings, will be instrumental in getting the message out to the public (Kennedy, Polivka, and Chaudry 1999). As effective clinicians of specialized care, they will be in demand for mental health services and preventive programs.

Society is becoming aware of the sharp increase in violent episodes in the community and in the home. Violence is a public health problem that will take an integrated community response to make homes, schools, workplaces, and public space safe from violent attacks (U.S. Department of Health and Human Services, U.S. Public Health Service 1998). Such a response requires collaboration among the health care, legal, social, and political constituencies. Nurses should seek opportunities to be advocates for violence prevention. They can play leadership roles in community initiatives that intimately involve the mental health of individuals and families.

Emerging issues and trends provide the impetus for lifelong learning by psychiatric-mental health nurses (Delaney et al. 1999; Pelletier et al. 1999). It is clear in this era of profound change that the challenge for these nurses is to retain the core values of psychiatric nursing, such as the centrality of the nurse-patient relationship and the inherent meaning of behavior (Forchuck et al. 2000). At the same time, they must integrate the new knowledge and skills that are required to provide the highest level of quality care. The scope and standards of psychiatric-mental health clinical practice contained in this document are intended to be anchors for the provision of quality mental health care as nurses journey in the turbulent currents of tomorrow's health care environment.

SCOPE OF PRACTICE FOR
PSYCHIATRIC MENTAL-HEALTH NURSING

This scope of practice statement and these standards are established by the profession and published through the auspices of the professional association for nurses, the ANA. They represent the profession's position on the practice of nursing within the specialty of psychiatric-mental health nursing.

Registered nurses are licensed and approved to practice by their individual states. Requirements for recognition for practice and for the performance of certain role functions vary from state to state. Each state has its own rules and regulations governing entry practice, advanced practice, and license renewal. Some states are exploring methods such as interstate compacts to facilitate movement of registered nurses from one state to another. Some states may require proof of additional credentials such as specific formal or continuing education course work or some type of certification to approve registered nurses to perform certain functions or to assume certain roles or titles.

There is certification in psychiatric-mental health nursing available at both the generalist and specialist levels. Some states and some payment sources may require proof of additional credentials for practice above the entry level. Various add-on options for certification are available in the specialty both in nursing and in other related categories such as marriage and family therapy and addictions counseling. Requirements set for credentialing are the purview of the credentialing body and not necessarily considered by the profession as requisites for practice.

Psychiatric-mental health nursing is the diagnosis and treatment of human responses to actual or potential mental health problems. Psychiatric-mental health nursing is a specialized area of nursing practice, employing the wide range of explanatory theories of, and research on, human behavior as its science, and purposeful use of self as its art.

Psychiatric-mental health nursing involves the delivery of comprehensive primary mental health care in a variety of settings. *Primary mental health care* is defined as the continuous and comprehensive services necessary for promotion of optimal mental health; the prevention of mental illness; health maintenance; management of, and referral for, mental and physical health problems; the diagnosis and treatment of mental disorders and their sequelae; and rehabilitation (Haber and Billings 1993). Psychiatric-mental health nursing is necessarily holistic and considers the needs and strengths of the individual, family, group, and community.

Diagnosis of human responses to actual or potential mental health problems involves the application of theory to human phenomena, through the processes of assessment, diagnosis, outcomes identification, planning, intervention or treatment, and evaluation. Theories and research relevant to psychiatric-mental health nursing are derived from various sources, including those from nursing, biological, cultural, environmental, psychological, and sociological sciences. These theories and research provide a basis for psychiatric-mental health nursing practice.

The psychiatric-mental health nurse's assessment is a synthesis of the information obtained from interviews, behavioral observations, and other available data from which a diagnosis is derived and validated with the patient, when appropriate. The psychiatric-mental health nurse uses diagnoses and standard classifications of mental disorders, such as North American Nursing Diagnosis Association (NANDA 1999), *The Diagnostic and Statistical Manual of Mental Disorders* of the American Psychiatric Association (American Psychiatric Association 1994), or the *International Classification of Diseases* (WHO, 1993) to develop a treatment plan based on assessment data and theoretical premises. The nurse then selects and implements interventions directed toward a patient's response to an actual or potential health problem. The nurse periodically evaluates the patient outcome and revises the plan of care to achieve optimal results. When possible, the psychiatric-mental health nurse chooses interventions and outcomes from recognized classification systems. Such classification systems enhance communication and permit the data to be used for research purposes.

The phenomena of concern for psychiatric-mental health nursing include actual or potential mental health problems of patients pertaining to

- the maintenance of optimal health and well-being and the prevention of mental illness.

- self-care limitations or impaired functioning related to mental, emotional, and physiological distress.

- deficits in the functioning of significant biological, emotional, and cognitive systems.

- emotional stress or crisis related to illness, pain, disability, and loss.

- self-concept and body image changes, developmental issues, life process changes, and end-of-life issues.

- problems related to emotions such as anxiety, anger, powerlessness, confusion, fear, sadness, loneliness, and grief.

- physical symptoms that occur along with altered psychological functioning.

- psychological symptoms that occur along with altered physiological functioning.

- alterations in thinking, perceiving, symbolizing, communicating, and decision-making.

- difficulties in relating to others.

- behaviors and mental states that indicate the patient is a danger to self or others or has a severe disability.

- symptom management, side effects/toxicities associated with self-administered drugs, psychopharmacological intervention, and other aspects of the treatment regimen.

- interpersonal, organizational, sociocultural, spiritual, or environmental circumstances or events which have an effect on the mental and emotional well-being of the individual, family, or community.

Psychiatric-Mental Health Nursing Clinical Practice Activities

Psychiatric-mental health nurses, in a variety of mental health settings, plan and implement services to meet patients' needs for a stable emotional and social support system. The psychiatric-mental health nurse works with individuals, families, groups, and communities to assess mental health needs, develop diagnoses, identify outcomes, and plan, implement, and evaluate nursing care. Planning and implementing these services focuses on meeting patients' needs for a stable emotional and social support system. The psychiatric-mental health nurse practices the use of self as a therapeutic resource through one-to-one or group interactions, in structured or informal sessions, and in the physical as well as the psychosocial aspects of care.

Levels of Psychiatric-Mental Health Clinical Nursing Practice

Psychiatric-mental health nurses are registered nurses who are educationally prepared in nursing and licensed to practice in their individual states. Psychiatric-mental health nurses are qualified for specialty practice at two levels—basic and advanced. These levels are differentiated by educational preparation, complexity of practice, and performance of certain nursing functions (Society for Education and Research for Psychiatric-Mental Health Nursing 1996).

Basic Level

Registered nurses at the basic level have completed a nursing program and passed the state licensure examination. Registered nurses who practice in psychiatric-mental health settings work as staff nurses, case managers, nurse managers, and in other nursing roles in the psychiatric-mental health field.

The psychiatric-mental health registered nurse (RN-PMH) is a registered nurse who has a baccalaureate degree in nursing, has worked in the field of psychiatric-mental health nursing for a minimum of two years, and demonstrates competency in the skills of psychiatric-mental health nursing identified in this document. Both the registered nurse and psychiatric-mental health registered nurse work at the basic level and are responsible for adhering to the scope and standards of psychiatric-mental health clinical nursing practice delineated in this document.

Basic Level Practice

Basic level psychiatric-mental health nursing practice is characterized by interventions that promote and foster health, assess dysfunction, assist patients to regain or improve their coping abilities, maximize strengths, and prevent further disability. These interventions focus on psychiatric-mental health patients and include health promotion and health maintenance, intake screening and evaluation, case management, provision of a therapeutic environment (e.g., milieu therapy), monitoring patients and assisting them with self-care activities, administering and monitoring psychobiological treatment regimens (including prescribed psychopharmacological agents and their effects), health teaching, counseling and crisis care, and psychiatric rehabilitation.

Health Promotion and Health Maintenance. The psychiatric-mental health nurse emphasizes health promotion and health maintenance reflecting nursing's long-standing concern for individual, family, group, and community well-being. The nurse conducts health assessments, targets situations that put people at risk, and initiates interventions such as assertiveness training, stress management, parenting classes, and health teaching, in addition to targeting potential complications related to symptoms of physical and mental illness and adverse treatment effects.

Intake Screening and Evaluation. At the point of an individual patient's entry into the mental health system, the psychiatric-mental health nurse performs intake screening and evaluation including biopsychosocial assessments, makes triage decisions, and facilitates the patient's movement into appropriate services. Data collection at the point of contact involves observational and investigative activities, which are guided by the nurse's knowledge of human behavior and the principles of the psychiatric interviewing process. The psychiatric-mental health nurse considers biophysical, psychological, social, cultural, spiritual, economic, and environmental aspects of the patient's life situation to gain an understanding of the problem as it has been experienced and to plan the kind of assistance that is indicated. The nurse is responsible for recognizing areas where additional clinical data are needed and referring the patient for more specialized testing and evaluation.

Case Management. Case management is a clinical component of the psychiatric-mental health nurse's role in both inpatient and outpatient settings. Nurses who are functioning in the case manager role support the patient's highest level of functioning through interventions that are designed to enhance self-sufficiency and progress toward optimal health. These interventions may include risk assessment, supportive counseling, problem solving, teaching, medication and health status monitoring, comprehensive care planning, and linkage to, and identification and coordination of, various other health and human services.

Milieu Therapy. The psychiatric-mental health nurse utilizes the human and other resources of institutional and community-based programs to foster the restoration or acquisition of the patients' skills and abilities. A key idea in milieu therapy is that any aspect of the environment can exert a major influence on behavior, facilitating or impeding the individual's potential for growth and change. On behalf of individual patients, the psychiatric-mental health nurse assesses and develops the therapeutic potential of a given setting by attending to a wide range of factors such as the physical environment, the social structure and interaction processes, and the culture of the setting.

Promotion of Self-Care Activities. A major dimension of direct nursing care functions within the therapeutic milieu involves self-care activities of daily living. There are many examples of nursing care that take advantage of the learning potential inherent in the daily life cycle. These include teaching medication regimen and symptom management, fostering recreational activities, and facilitating development in the practical skills of community life, such as shopping, workplace skills, and using public transportation. By comforting, guiding, and setting limits, the psychiatric-mental health nurse can make use of patients' experiences of daily living to help them to move from dependent to independent and interdependent modes of behavior.

Psychobiological Interventions. Another dimension of psychiatric-mental health nursing derives from the understanding and application of psychobiological knowledge bases for psychiatric-mental health nursing care. The nurse's distinctive contribution rests in the ability to evaluate holistically and treat patient responses to actual and potential health problems. The psychiatric-mental health nurse employs psychobiological interventions, which include various emergency procedures in addition to standard nursing measures such as relaxation techniques, other complementary therapies, nutrition/diet regulation, exercise and rest schedules, and other somatic treatments. The psychiatric-mental health nurse monitors patient responses to all psychobiological interventions and the overall treatment program, including such activities as the administration and management of medications, recovery from electroconvulsive therapy, and implementation of other treatment regimens.

A frequent component of services is the psychiatric-mental health nurse's support and oversight of the patient's pharmacotherapeutic treatment. As a result of monitoring the patient's response to these interventions, the nurse is frequently in a position to identify problems or side effects, report these to the prescribing clinician, and advocate for necessary adjustments in treatment. Medication education and monitoring may be provided on an individual or group basis. The aim is to teach patients about their medications, invite their questions, listen to their concerns, and assist them in dealing with practical problems related to side effects and other difficulties they may encounter when continuing a prescribed medication regimen in unsupervised settings. These activities also include the use of nonprescribed, over-the-counter medications and supplements.

Complementary interventions include a range of modalities, such as diet/nutrition regulation, relaxation techniques, therapeutic touch, mindfulness meditation, and guided imagery. In utilizing these therapies, the psychiatric-mental health nurse applies understanding of the modality and its potential therapeutic benefits, and is vigilant in responding to any untoward reactions.

Health Teaching. Psychiatric-mental health nurses combine knowledge of the principles of teaching and learning, with knowledge of health and illness, as they integrate health teaching throughout their work with individuals, families, and community groups. The need for health teaching relates to biological, pharmacological, physical, sociocultural, or psychological aspects of the learner's care. Selection of particular formal and informal learning methods depends on identified needs and learning outcomes. Nurses recognize that experiential learning opportunities are particularly important in developing appropriate coping skills and an understanding of mental health problems. Constructive role modeling by the psychiatric-mental health nurse is an inherent part of the teaching function.

Counseling. In psychiatric-mental health nursing, the aim of counseling is to focus specifically, and for a limited period of time, with a patient, family, or group, on a problem representing an immediate difficulty related to health or well-being. The patient's issue is investigated using a supportive problem-solving approach, so that the experience may be understood more fully, integrated with other life experiences, and promote constructive personal change.

Crisis Care. Psychiatric-mental health nurses provide crisis intervention, stabilization, and direct counseling services to persons in crisis as individual needs arise, or as members of crisis teams. Crisis care is a short-term therapeutic process that focuses on the resolution of an immediate crisis or emergency through the use of supportive problem solving and mobilization of personnel, family, and/or environmental resources.

Psychiatric Rehabilitation. Psychiatric rehabilitation nursing practice focuses on improving an individual's quality of life by facilitating symptom management and by promoting relapse prevention. Approaches are designed to strengthen self-care skills, decrease hospitalization rates, and promote integration into community life. Within a rehabilitation and recovery context, the nurse-patient relationship is viewed as a collaborative partnership. Interventions are focused on the development of life skills and the identification and use of environmental supports (Palmer-Erbs and Anthony 1995).

Advanced Level Psychiatric-Mental Health Nursing Practice

The advanced practice registered nurse in psychiatric-mental health (APRN-PMH) is a licensed registered nurse who is educationally prepared either as a clinical nurse specialist or a nurse practitioner at least at the master's degree level in the specialty of psychiatric-mental health nursing. The nurse's graduate level preparation is distinguished by a depth of knowledge of theory and practice, validated experience in clinical practice, and competence in advanced clinical nursing skills. The APRN-PMH focuses clinical practice on persons with diagnosed psychiatric disorders, or those vulnerable individuals or populations at risk of mental health disorders. The APRN-PMH applies knowledge, skills, and experience autonomously to complex psychiatric-mental health problems and the promotion of mental health within our society. The APRN-PMH collaborates with and refers to other professionals as the patient's needs and the nurse's practice focus dictates.

The advanced practice role and function descriptions defined within this document are intended to apply specifically and exclusively to the specialty area of psychiatric-mental health nursing. APRNs (clinical nurse specialists and nurse practitioners) providing physical health care to the population at large or in other patient groups, should refer to the appropriate nursing standards that apply to that practice.

The scope of practice in psychiatric-mental health nursing is continually expanding as the context of practice, the need for patient access to holistic care, and the various scientific and nursing knowledge bases evolve. In addition to the long-standing role of the APRN-PMH as a psychotherapist, the United States Congress and many state legislatures have acknowledged the unique competency of the APRN-PMH in the delivery of mental health services by passing legislation, which also makes the APRN-PMH eligible for prescriptive authority, inpatient admission privileges, third-party reimbursement, and other specific privileges.

It is within the scope of practice of APRN-PMH nurses, whether prepared as clinical specialists or as nurse practitioners, to provide primary mental health care to patients seeking mental health services in a wide range of delivery settings. Primary mental health care involves overall health promotion, universal, selective, and preventive mental health interventions (Mrazek and Hagerty 1994), general health teaching, health screening, and appropriate referral for treatment of general or complex health problems and a specialization in the evaluation and management of those with mental disorders and those at risk for them, including psychiatric rehabilitation (Haber and Billings 1995).

Although the APRN-PMH can perform all aspects of the role functions of the psychiatric-mental health nurse at the basic level of practice, the professional parameters of psychiatric-mental health nursing at the advanced level include the complete delivery of direct primary mental health care services including, but not limited to

- carrying out health promotion activities including general health teaching.

- designing and conducting mental illness preventive interventions.

- conducting health screening and evaluation.
- eliciting a history appropriate to the patient, presentation, and setting.
- completing a health assessment/examination.
- formulating differential diagnoses based on clinical findings.
- ordering, conducting, and interpreting pertinent laboratory and diagnostic studies and procedures.
- formulating, implementing, and evaluating an outcome-based treatment plan.
- conducting individual, family, group, and network psychotherapy.
- directing and providing home health services to mental health patients.
- prescribing, monitoring, managing, and evaluating psychopharmacological and related medications.
- providing integrated mental health services in general health settings.
- facilitating psychiatric rehabilitation.

This holistic practice includes a responsibility for collaboration with patients, families and other clinicians, and referral for services which fall outside the nurse's practice parameters. The practice of the APRN-PMH is limited to the provision of primary mental health care services to those at risk for mental disorders or presently in need of psychiatric-mental health services. This practice does not extend to the provision of primary care services. If the APRN-PMH is also educationally prepared as either as a clinical nurse specialist or nurse practitioner in a different specialty, the APRN-PMH is qualified to provide services to those other patient populations. Although many primary care clinicians treat some symptoms of mental disorders, the APRN-PMH provides the full range of services that comprise primary mental health care.

Each individual ARN-PMH is not expected to perform every function identified within the scope of practice for advanced psychiatric-mental health nursing. All nurses are accountable for practicing in accordance with state law and within the limits of their knowledge, skills, and abilities, taking into account what is therapeutic for each individual patient. Even though a function is within the nurse's scope of practice, the nurse may decide to refer that aspect of care to another clinician.

The APRN-PMH is professionally qualified to assume autonomous responsibility for the clinical role functions. Such nurses are accountable for their own practices and are prepared to perform services independent of any other discipline in the full range of delivery settings. The educational preparation of advanced practice psychiatric-mental health nurses in both the biological and social sciences gives them a unique ability to differentiate various aspects of the patient's functioning and to make appropriate judgments about the need for interventions, referral, or consultation with other clinicians. Proficiency in the art and science of advanced practice psychiatric-mental health nursing is an outgrowth of advanced, specialized educational experience and of activities to refine and update knowledge and skills through practice, continuing education, and the voluntary use of consultation and collaboration with other clinicians.

Additional functions practiced by the APRN-PMH include the advanced level practice of psychopharmacological interventions, complementary interventions, various forms of psychotherapy, community interventions, case management, consultation-liaison, clinical supervision, and expanded advocacy activities.

Psychopharmacology interventions include the prescription of pharmacological agents and the ordering and interpretation of diagnostic and laboratory testing. In utilizing any psychobiological interventions, including the prescription of psychoactive medications, the APRN-PMH intentionally seeks specific therapeutic responses, anticipates any side effects, safeguards against adverse drug interactions, and is alert for unintended or toxic responses.

Psychotherapy interventions include all generally accepted methods of brief or long-term therapy, specifically including individual therapy (e.g., insight therapy, behavioral therapy, goal- or solution-oriented therapy, relationship therapy, cognitive therapy, and play and other expressive therapies), group therapy, couple/marital therapy, and family therapy. *Psychotherapy* denotes a formally structured contractual relationship between the therapist and patient(s) for the explicit purpose of effecting negotiated outcomes. It is a treatment approach to mental disorders that is intended to alleviate emotional distress, reverse or change maladaptive behavior, and facilitate personal growth and development. It involves a therapeutic contract, which is structured with the patient at the beginning of the relationship. Included in the terms of the contract are such elements as purpose, time, place, fees, the individuals participating, confidentiality, and access to emergency after-hours assistance. To ensure quality, the therapist continually scrutinizes the therapy sessions in relation to the content, process, and rationales for therapeutic judgments and actions.

Community interventions occur at the macro-system level in community mental health and other environments such as occupational or primary care settings. In community focus, the APRN-PMH analyzes the health needs of populations and designs programs, which target at-risk groups. Community interventions include attention to cultural, developmental, and environmental factors that foster health and prevent mental illness.

Case management activities facilitate the use of health care and other appropriate resources to promote the health of the patient. In addition to basic level case management activities, the APRN-PMH uses population-specific nursing knowledge coupled with research, knowledge of the legal system related to mental health, and expertise in supportive psychotherapy to obtain services needed for the patient, regardless of the setting. The APRN-PMH analyzes barriers to care and identifies system improvements needed. The result is the mobilization of therapeutic resources needed by the patient and the maximization of positive outcomes. Case management activities may be used with a single client or for populations such as the seriously and persistently mentally ill.

Consultation-liaison activities take place in general (nonpsychiatric) health care arenas such as hospitals, extended care facilities, rehabilitation centers, and outpatient clinics where the APRN-PMH practices consultation-liaison nursing to provide mental health specialist consultation or direct care psychiatric-mental health nursing services. The clinical aspect of this role ranges from mental health promotion to illness rehabilitation. In consultation-liaison activities, the APRN-PMH focuses on the emotional, spiritual, developmental, cognitive, and behavioral responses of patients who enter any setting of the health care system with actual or potential physiological dysfunction (client-centered consultation). This psychiatric-mental health consultation may include consultee-centered consultation with nurses and clinicians in other specialty areas to increase their biopsychosocial knowledge and skills. Such consultation may also assist them to recognize and manage their own reactions to patients that, undetected and unaddressed, could adversely affect their patient care. Psychiatric-mental health consultation may also include assessment and recommendations for action focusing on the health care delivery organization as the client (administrative consultation) (Caplan and Caplan 1993).

Clinical supervisory activities are those in which the APRN-PMH provides clinical supervision to assist other PMH clinicians in further developing their clinical practice skills, in meeting the standard requirement for ongoing peer consultation, and in providing essential peer supervision. This is an educative and professional growth development process, not a staff performance evaluation. Through education, preparation, and clinical experience, the APRN-PMH is qualified to provide clinical supervision at the request of other mental health clinicians and clinician-trainees. The clinical supervisor is expected to provide direct care to selected patients and serve as a clinical role model as well as a clinical consultant.

Psychiatric-Mental Health Nursing Clinical Practice Settings

There are two principal arrangements for the clinical practice of psychiatric-mental health nursing: organized health care settings and self-employment. Nurses who work within organized settings are paid for their services on a salaried, contractual, or fee-for-service basis. The settings and arrangements for psychiatric-mental health nursing practice vary widely in purpose, type, location, and the auspices under which they are operated.

Community-based Care

Some nurses enter the social environments that are integral parts of people's daily lives—homes, schools, and work sites—to provide mental health services providing primary mental health care and preserving the supports that facilitate family and social network functioning. Psychiatric-mental health nurses provide care within the community as an effective method of responding to the mental health needs of individuals, families, or groups. *Community-based care* refers to care delivered in partnerships with patients in homes, worksites, halfway houses, educational and judicial system programs, home-health agencies, employee assistance programs, mental health clinics, health maintenance organizations, primary care centers, shelters and clinics for the homeless, senior centers, emergency and crisis centers, day care shelters for battered women and children, soup kitchens, shelters for individuals with chronic mental illness, day care settings, residential treatment facilities, group homes for identified populations, nursing homes, foster care residences, and other community settings.

Psychiatric home health care is increasingly being used in some situations as an alternative to inpatient treatment. The patient and the family may be seen as needed to restabilize the patient's condition. Home health services may also be useful in medication management for patients who are prone to severe side effects or who need regular titration of their medications. The nurse may select the home visit as the most efficacious means of intervention by helping to stimulate the potential helping responses of family members or other significant persons. Efforts to help the family adapt to the re-entry of the discharged psychiatric patient into the home environment is another example of the nurse's function within the home setting. The psychiatric mental health nurse also may provide physical health care services.

Intermediate- and Long-term Care

Psychiatric-mental health nurses practice effectively in a range of intermediate- and long-term care settings that exist for treatment and support of those with severe and persistent mental disorders. These includes day- and night-care services, residential care facilities, rehabilitation settings, and therapeutic foster care as well as other innovative service delivery programs. Psychiatric-mental health nurses continue to practice in psychiatric treatment settings such as general hospitals, psychiatric units of community hospitals, centers for detoxification and the treatment of chemical dependence, psychiatric rehabilitation facilities, private inpatient settings, the publicly funded hospital system, and correctional facilities. An important focus for the nurse is to assist in the patient's transition from the institutional to the community setting.

Telehealth

The psychiatric mental health nurse may utilize electronic means of communication (telephone consultation, faxing, computers, electronic mail, image transmission, interactive video sessions) to establish and maintain a therapeutic relationship with a patient by creating an alternative sense of the nursing presence that may or may not occur in "real" time. This modality is identified as the practice of *telehealth*, which is the removal of time and distance barriers for the delivery of health care services and related health care activities through telecommunications technologies (Milholland 1997). It is an expanded means of communication that promotes access to health care. The technology is also being used in educational programs and research (ANA 1998).

Nurses using telehealth technology deliver direct health services in health care facilities, clinics, private offices, and the home. Because it can cross state and national boundaries, telehealth is to be practiced in accordance with all applicable state, federal, and international laws and regulations.

The nurse should use practice and clinical guidelines for telehealth that are based on empirical evidence and professional consensus. Particular attention is directed to the confidentiality of telehealth encounters, informed consent, documentation, the maintenance of records, and the integrity of the transmitted information. The nurse using telehealth technology is competent in the various hardware and software being utilized.

Self-employment

Self-employed APRN-PMHs offer direct services in solo private practice and group practice settings, or through contracts with employee assistance programs, health maintenance organizations, managed care companies, preferred provider organizations, industry health departments, home health care agencies, or other service delivery arrangements. In these settings, the APRN-PMH provides primary mental health care to patients in the nurse's caseload. The APRN-PMH in the consultation-liaison role may also contract for consultation services focused on the needs of the organization and its staff, or on the needs of patients in a variety of health care settings. These self-employed nurses also may form nurse-owned corporations or organizations that can compete with other provider groups for mental health service contracts with industries or employers.

Subspecialization

Subspecialization within psychiatric-mental health nursing has emerged based on current and anticipated societal needs for a specific category of patients. This subspecialization may be organized according to a developmental period (e.g., child and adolescent, adult, geriatric) (ANA 1985), a specific mental/emotional disorder (e.g., addiction; depression; severe, persistent mental illness), a particular practice focus (e.g., community, group, couple, family, individuals), and/or a specific role or function (e.g., case management, psychiatric consultation-liaison). Subspecialty categories are not mutually exclusive but provide a matrix within which the parameters of subspecialization are defined.

Formal or continuing education, additional training and experience, and the individual nurse's judgment about readiness to work with a particular situation or patient population constitute appropriate preparation for subspecialty practice. For example, psychiatric-mental health nurses experienced with patients with severe mental illness in hospitals settings may elect to refocus their practice to patients in a geropsychiatric day treatment program. APRN-PMHs in adult psychiatric-mental health nursing may appropriately work with children as part of a family approach, either in family therapy or adjunctively in the treatment of the child's parents. Similarly, APRN-PMHs working in child and adolescent psychiatric-mental health nursing may see adults (e.g., parents or guardians) in therapy. In each of these situations, it is the responsibility of the individual nurse to develop the knowledge and skills required to provide services to the subspecialty group.

Advocacy and Social Responsibility

Advocacy

Because of nursing's strong commitment to the health, welfare, and safety of the patient, the nurse must be aware of any activity that places the rights or well-being of the patient in jeopardy and take appropriate action on the patient's behalf. In clinical practice, the nurse-advocate vigilantly protects the rights of patients and speaks for those who, for whatever reason, cannot speak for themselves. In addition, functioning as advocates, nurses are engaging in public speaking, writing articles for the popular press, and lobbying their congressional representatives on behalf of better mental health and psychiatric care for all persons.

Expanded Advocacy Activities

A particularly important dimension of the clinical role of psychiatric-mental health nurses is that of the advocate and policy influencer/maker. Nurses have a long history of supporting the cause of one of the most neglected constituencies—persons with mental illness. Ongoing political activism is necessary to ensure that the rights of those with mental illness are protected. Some APRN-PMH nurses are influencing public policy by assuming leadership positions in government agencies at the local, state, and federal levels, or by running for public office. Others are joining consumer and professional groups' campaigns to demystify mental illness, abolish the stigma so often attached to it, and achieve parity between mental and physical illness health care coverage.

Social Responsibility

Psychiatric-mental health nursing includes concern for sociocultural factors that adversely affect the mental health of population groups and the design of activities that can ameliorate these problems. Involvement with community planning boards, advisory groups, paraprofessionals, and other key people is an important means by which nurses can mobilize the community's resources and bring about changes that address the mental health needs of particular population groups.

Psychiatric-Mental Health Nursing Ethics

Nursing's respect for the patient's dignity, autonomy, cultural beliefs, and privacy is of particular concern in psychiatric-mental health nursing practice. The nurse serves as an advocate for the patient and is obliged to demonstrate nonjudgmental and nondiscriminatory attitudes and behaviors that are sensitive to patient diversity. An essential aspect of the patient's response is the right to exercise personal choice about participation in proposed treatments. The responsible use of the nurse's authority respects the patient's freedom to choose among existing alternatives and facilitates awareness of resources available to assist with decision making. However, as mental health law recognizes, there are situations in which mental health professionals must decide to set aside the patient's choices for the sake of the patient's own safety or for the safety of others. In these situations, the psychiatric-mental health nurse strives to protect the rights of the patient as much as possible, and works to ensure that the patient's right to choose is restricted only as necessary.

Nurses working with psychiatric-mental health patients are prepared to recognize the special nature of the clinician-patient relationship and take steps to assure therapeutic relationships are conducted in a manner that adheres to the mandates stipulated in the ANA Code for Nurses (ANA 1985). Unethical behavior (e.g., omission of informed consent, breach of confidentiality, coercion, boundary infringement) and illegal acts can increase the patient's vulnerability and demand special vigilance on the part of the psychiatric-mental health nurse.

STANDARDS OF CARE

"Standards of Care" pertain to professional nursing activities that are demonstrated by the nurse through the nursing process. These involve assessment, diagnosis, outcome identification, planning, implementation, and evaluation. The nursing process is the foundation of clinical decision making and encompasses all significant action taken by nurses in providing developmentally and culturally relevant psychiatric mental-health care to all patients.

Standard I. Assessment

The psychiatric-mental health nurse collects patient health data.

Rationale

The assessment interview, which requires linguistically and culturally effective communication skills, interviewing, behavioral observation, record review, and comprehensive assessment of the patient and relevant systems, enables the psychiatric-mental health nurse to make sound clinical judgments and plan appropriate interventions with the patient.

Measurement Criteria

1. The priority of data collection is determined by the patient's immediate condition or need.

2. The data may include but are not limited to the patient's

   a. ability to remain safe and not be a danger to oneself and others.

   b. central complaint, symptoms, or focus or concern.

   c. physical, developmental, cognitive, mental, and emotional health status.

   d. demographic profile and history of health patterns, illnesses, and past treatments.

   e. family, social, cultural, race, ethnicity, and community systems.

f. daily activities, functional health status, substance use, health habits, and social roles, including work and sexual functioning.

g. interpersonal relationships, communication skills, and coping patterns.

h. spiritual, religious, or philosophical beliefs and values.

i. economic, political, legal, and environmental factors affecting health.

j. significant support systems and community resources, both available and underutilized.

k. health beliefs and practices.

l. knowledge, satisfaction, and motivation to change, related to health.

m. strengths and competencies that can be used to promote health.

n. current and past medications, including prescribed and over-the-counter.

o. medication interactions and history of side effects.

p. complementary therapies used to treat health and mental illness.

q. other contributing factors that influence health and mental health.

3. Pertinent data are collected from multiple sources using various developmentally and culturally appropriate assessment techniques, standardized instruments, and diagnostic and laboratory tests. Multiple sources of assessment data can include not only the patient, but also family, social network, other health care clinicians, past and current medical records, and community agencies and systems (with consideration of the patient's confidentiality).

4. The patient, significant others, and interdisciplinary team members are involved in the assessment process and data analysis.

5. The patient and significant others are informed of their respective roles and responsibilities in the assessment process and data analysis.

6. The assessment process is systematic and ongoing.

7. The data collection is based on clinical judgment to ensure that relevant and necessary data are collected.

8. The database is synthesized, prioritized, and documented in a retrievable form.

Standard II. Diagnosis

The psychiatric-mental health nurse analyzes the assessment data in determining diagnoses.

Rationale

The basis for providing psychiatric-mental health nursing care is the recognition and identification of patterns of response to actual or potential psychiatric illnesses, mental health problems, and potential comorbid physical illnesses.

Measurement Criteria

1. Diagnoses and potential problem statements are derived from assessment data.

2. Interpersonal, systematic, or environmental circumstances that affect the mental well-being of the individual, family, or community are identified.

3. The diagnosis is based on an accepted framework that supports the psychiatric-mental health nursing knowledge and judgment used in analyzing the data.

4. Diagnoses conform to accepted classifications systems, such as NANDA or other nursing classifications, *International Classification of Diseases and Statistical Manual of Mental Diseases* (WHO 1993), and *The Diagnostic and Statistical Manual of Mental Disorders–IV Edition* (APA 1994) used in the practice setting.

5. Diagnoses and risk factors are discussed and verified with the patient, significant others, and other health care clinicians when appropriate and possible.

6. Diagnoses identify actual or potential psychiatric illness and mental health problems of patients.

7. Diagnoses and clinical impressions are documented in a manner that facilitates the identification of patient outcomes and their use in the plan of care and research.

Standard III. Outcome Identification

The psychiatric-mental health nurse identifies expected outcomes individualized to the patient.

Rationale

Within the context of providing nursing care, the ultimate goal is to influence mental health outcomes and improve the patient's health status.

Measurement Criteria

1. Expected outcomes are derived from the diagnoses.

2. Expected outcomes are patient-oriented, evidence-based, therapeutically sound, realistic, attainable, and cost-effective.

3. Expected outcomes are documented as measurable goals using standard classifications when available.

4. Expected outcomes are formulated by the nurse and the patient, significant others, and interdisciplinary team members, when possible.

5. Expected outcomes are realistic in relation to the patient's present and potential capabilities and quality of life.

6. Expected outcomes are identified with consideration of the associated benefits and costs.

7. Expected outcomes estimate a time for attainment.

8. Expected outcomes provide direction for continuity of care.

9. Expected outcomes reflect current scientific knowledge in mental health care.

10. Expected outcomes serve as a record of change in the patient's health status.

Standard IV. Planning

The psychiatric-mental health nurse develops a plan of care that is negotiated among the patient, nurse, family, and health care team and prescribes evidence-based interventions to attain expected outcomes.

Rationale

A plan of care is used to guide therapeutic interventions systematically, document progress, and achieve the expected patient outcomes.

Measurement Criteria

1. The plan is individualized according to the patient's characteristics, needs, health problems and condition, and

   a. identifies priorities of care in relation to expected outcomes.

   b. identifies effective interventions to achieve outcomes.

   c. specifies evidence-based interventions that reflect current best practices and research.

   d. reflects the patient's motivation, health beliefs, and functional capabilities.

   e. includes an educational program related to the patient's health problems, stress management, treatment regimen, relapse prevention, self-care activities, and quality of life.

   f. indicates responsibilities of the nurse, the patient, the family and other significant persons, and the interdisciplinary team members in implementing the plan.

   g. gives direction to patient care activities designated by the nurse to the family, significant others, and other care clinicians.

      h. provides the appropriate referral and case management to ensure continuity of care.

      i. considers the benefits and costs of interventions in relation to outcomes.

2. The plan is developed in collaboration with the patient, significant others, and the interdisciplinary team members, when appropriate.

3. The plan is documented in a format that allows modification, as necessary, interdisciplinary access to its information, and retrieval of data for analysis and research.

Standard V. Implementation

The psychiatric-mental health nurse implements the interventions identified in the plan of care.

Rationale

In implementing the plan of care, psychiatric-mental health nurses use a wide range of interventions designed to prevent mental and physical illness, and promote, maintain, and restore mental and physical health. Psychiatric-mental health nurses select interventions according to their level of practice. At the basic level, nurses may select counseling milieu therapy, promotion of self-care activities, intake screening and evaluation, psychobiological interventions, health teaching, case management, health promotion and health maintenance, crisis intervention, community-based care, psychiatric home health care, telehealth, and a variety of other approaches to meet the mental health needs of patients. In addition to the intervention options available to the basic-level psychiatric-mental health nurse, at the advanced level the APRN-PMH may provide consultation, engage in psychotherapy, and prescribe pharmacological agents in accordance with state statutes or regulations.

Measurement Criteria

1. A therapeutic nurse-patient relationship is established and maintained throughout treatment.

2. Interventions are based on research when available.

3. Interventions are implemented according to the established plan of care.

4. Interventions are performed according to the psychiatric-mental health nurse's level of education and practice.

5. Interventions are performed in a safe, timely, ethical, and appropriate manner.

6. Interventions are modified based on continued assessment of the patient's response to treatment and other clinical indicators of effectiveness.

7. Interventions are documented in a format that is related to patient outcomes, accessible to the interdisciplinary team, and retrievable for future data analysis and research.

Standard Va. Counseling

The psychiatric-mental health nurse uses counseling interventions to assist patients in improving or regaining their previous coping abilities, fostering mental health, and preventing mental illness and disability.

Measurement Criteria

1. Counseling promotes the patient's personal and social integration.

2. Counseling reinforces healthy behaviors and interaction patterns, and helps the patient modify or discontinue unhealthy ones.

3. The documentation of counseling interventions, including communication and interviewing techniques, problem-solving activities, crisis intervention, stress management, support groups, relaxation techniques, assertiveness training, substance abuse counseling, conflict resolution, and behavior modification, is completed.

Standard Vb. Milieu Therapy

The psychiatric-mental health nurse provides, structures, and maintains a therapeutic environment in collaboration with the patient and other health care clinicians.

Measurement Criteria

1. The patient is familiarized with the physical environment, the schedule of activities, and the norms and rules that govern behavior and activities of daily living, as applicable.

2. Current knowledge of the effects of the environment on the patient is used to guide nursing actions and provide a safe environment.

3. The therapeutic environment is designed to make use of the physical environment, social structures, culture, and other available resources.

4. Therapeutic communication among patients and staff supports an effective milieu.

5. Specific activities are selected that meet the patient's physical and mental health needs.

6. Limits of any kind (e.g., restriction of privileges, restraint, seclusion, timeout) are used in a humane manner, are the least restrictive necessary, and are employed only as needed to ensure the safety of the patient and of others.

7. The patient is given information about the need for limits and the conditions necessary for removal of the restriction, as appropriate.

Standard Vc. Promotion of Self-Care Activities

The psychiatric-mental health nurse structures interventions around the patient's activities of daily living to foster self-care and mental and physical well-being.

Measurement Criteria

1. The self-care activities chosen are appropriate for the patient's physical and mental status as well as age, developmental level, gender, social orientation, ethnic/social background, and education.

2. The self-care interventions assist the patient in assuming responsibility for activities of daily living, including maintaining a medication regimen, engaging in health-promoting behaviors, and seeking therapeutic interventions when appropriate.

3. Self-care interventions are aimed at maintaining and improving the patient's functional status and quality of life.

Standard Vd. Psychobiological Interventions

The psychiatric-mental health nurse uses knowledge of psychobiological interventions and applies clinical skills to restore the patient's health and prevent further disability.

Measurement Criteria

1. Current research findings are applied to guide nursing actions related to psychopharmacology, other psychobiological therapies, and complementary therapies.

2. Psychopharmacological agents' intended actions, untoward or interactive effects, and therapeutic doses are monitored, as are blood levels, vital signs, and laboratory values where appropriate.

3. Nursing interventions are directed toward alleviating untoward effects of psychobiological interventions, when possible.

4. Nursing observations about the patient's response to psychobiological interventions are communicated to other health clinicians.

Standard Ve. Health Teaching

The psychiatric-mental health nurse, through health teaching, assists patients in achieving satisfying, productive, and healthy patterns of living.

Measurement Criteria

1. Health teaching is based on principles of learning.

2. Health teaching occurs on an individual basis or within a group context, depending on the information content and patient's ability.

3. Health teaching for the patient includes information about coping, interpersonal relations, mental health problems, mental disorders, social skills, and treatments and their effects on daily living, as well as information pertinent to physical status or developmental needs.

4. Constructive feedback and positive rewards reinforce the patient's learning.

5. Practice sessions, homework assignments, and experiential learning are used as needed.

6. Health teaching provides opportunities for the patient and significant others to question, discuss, and explore their thoughts and feelings about past, current, and projected use of therapies to make informed choices.

Standard Vf. Case Management

The psychiatric-mental health nurse provides case management to coordinate comprehensive health services and to ensure continuity of care.

Measurement Criteria

1. Case management services are based on a comprehensive approach to the patient's physical, mental, emotional, and social health problems and resource availability.

2. Case management services are provided in terms of the patient's needs, resources, and the accessibility, availability, quality, and cost-effectiveness of care.

3. Health-related services and more specialized care are negotiated on behalf of the patient with the appropriate agencies and providers as needed.

4. Relationships with agencies and providers are maintained throughout the patient's use of the health care services to ensure continuity of care.

Standard Vg. Health Promotion and Health Maintenance

The psychiatric-mental health nurse employs strategies and interventions to promote and maintain health and prevent mental illness.

Measurement Criteria

1. Health promotion and disease prevention strategies are based on knowledge of health beliefs, practices, evidence-based findings, and epidemiological principles, along with the social,

cultural, and political issues that affect mental health in an identified community.

2. Health promotion and disease prevention interventions are designed for patients identified as being at risk for mental health problems.

3. Consumer alliances and consumer participation are sought, as appropriate, in identifying mental health problems in the community and planning, implementing, and evaluating programs to address those problems.

4. Community resources are identified to assist consumers in using prevention and mental health care services appropriately.

5. Research findings are utilized to promote health and prevent mental illness.

The following interventions (Vh–Vj) may be performed only by the APRN-PMH.

Advanced Practice Interventions Vh–Vj

Standard Vh. Psychotherapy

The APRN-PMH uses individual, group, and family psychotherapy, and other therapeutic treatments to assist patients in preventing mental illness and disability, treating mental health disorders, and improving mental health status and functional abilities.

Measurement Criteria

1. The therapeutic contract with the patient is structured to include

   a. purpose, goals, and expected outcomes.

   b. time, place, and frequency of therapy.

   c. participants involved in therapy.

   d. confidentiality.

   e. availability and means of contacting therapist.

   f. responsibilities of both patient and therapist.

   g. fees and payment schedule.

2. Knowledge of personality theory, growth and development, psychology, neurobiology, psychopathology, social systems, small-group and family dynamics, stress and adaptation, and theories related to selected therapeutic methods is used, based on the patient's needs.

3. Therapeutic principles are used to understand and interpret the patient's emotions, thoughts, and behaviors.

4. The patient is helped to deal constructively with thoughts, emotions, and behaviors.

5. Increasing responsibility and independence are fostered in the patient to reinforce healthy behaviors and interactions.

6. In the therapist's absence, provision for care is arranged.

7. When it is determined that the provision of some aspect of physical care required by the patient would impair the therapist-patient relationship, referral for that care is made to another clinician.

Standard Vi. Prescriptive Authority and Treatment

The APRN-PMH uses prescriptive authority, procedures, and treatments in accordance with state and federal laws and regulations, to treat symptoms of psychiatric illness and improve functional health status.

Measurement Criteria

1. Psychiatric treatment interventions and procedures are prescribed according to the patient's mental health care needs and are evidence-based.

2. Procedures are used as needed in the delivery of comprehensive care.

3. Psychopharmacological agents are prescribed based on a knowledge of psychopathology, neurobiology, physiology, expected therapeutic actions, anticipated side effects, and courses of action, for unintended or toxic effects.

4. Pharmacological agents are prescribed based on clinical indicators of the patient's status, including the results of diagnostic and laboratory tests, as appropriate.

5. Intended effects and potential adverse effects of pharmacological and nonpharmacological treatments are monitored and treated as necessary.

6. Information about intended effects, potential adverse effects of the proposed prescription, and other treatment options, including no treatment, is provided to the patient.

7. Informed consent is obtained for treatment.

Standard Vj. Consultation

The APRN-PMH provides consultation to enhance the abilities of other clinicians to provide services for patients and effect change in the system.

Measurement Criteria

1. Consultation activities are based on models of consultation, systems principles, communication and interviewing techniques, problem-solving skills, change theories, and other theories indicated.

2. Consultation is initiated at the request of the consultee.

3. A working alliance, based on mutual respect and role responsibilities, is established with the patient or consultee.

4. Consultation recommendations are communicated in terms that facilitate understanding and involve the consultee in decision making.

5. Implementation of the system change or plan of care remains the consultee's responsibility.

Standard VI. Evaluation

The psychiatric-mental health nurse evaluates the patient's progress in attaining expected outcomes.

Rationale

Nursing care is a dynamic process involving change in the patient's health status over time, giving rise to the need for data, different diagnoses, and modifications in the plan of care. Therefore, evaluation is a continuous process of appraising the effect of nursing and the treatment regimen on the patient's health status and expected outcomes.

Measurement Criteria

1. Evaluation is systematic, ongoing, and criterion-based.

2. The patient, family or significant others, and other health care clinicians are involved in the evaluation process, as possible, to ascertain the patient's level of satisfaction with care and evaluate the benefits and costs associated with the treatment process.

3. The effectiveness of interventions in relation to outcomes is evaluated, using standardized methods as appropriate.

4. The patient's responses to treatment are documented in a format that is related to expected outcomes, accessible to the interdisciplinary team, and retrievable for data analysis and future research.

5. Ongoing assessment data are used to revise diagnoses, outcomes, and the plan of care as needed.

6. Revisions in the diagnoses, outcomes and plan of care are documented.

7. The revised plan provides for the continuity of care.

STANDARDS OF PROFESSIONAL PERFORMANCE

Standards of professional performance describe a competent level of behavior in the professional role, including activities related to quality of care, performance appraisal, education, collegiality, ethics, collaboration, research, and resource utilization. All psychiatric-mental health nurses are expected to engage in professional role activities appropriate to their education, position, and practice setting. Therefore, some standards or measurement criteria identify these activities.

Although standards of professional performance describe the roles of all professional nurses, there are many other responsibilities that are hallmarks of psychiatric-mental health nursing. These nurses should be self-directed and purposeful in seeking necessary knowledge and skills to enhance career goals. Other activities—such as membership in professional organizations, certification in specialty of advanced practice, continuing education, and further academic education—are desirable methods of enhancing the psychiatric-mental health nurse's professionalism.

Standard I. Quality of Care

The psychiatric-mental health nurse systematically evaluates the quality of care and effectiveness of psychiatric-mental health nursing practice.

Rationale

The dynamic nature of the mental health care environment and the growing body of psychiatric nursing knowledge and research provide both the impetus and the means for the psychiatric-mental heath nurse to be competent in clinical practice, to continue to develop professionally, and to improve the quality of patient care.

Measurement Criteria

1. The psychiatric-mental health nurse participates in safety and quality-of-care activities as appropriate to the nurse's

position, education, and practice environment. Such activities can include

a. identification of aspects of care important for quality monitoring; for example, functional status, symptom management and control, health behaviors and practices, safety, patient satisfaction, and quality of life.

b. utilization of existing, or development of new, quality indicators used to monitor the effectiveness of psychiatric-mental health nursing care.

c. collection of data to monitor quality and effectiveness of psychiatric-mental health nursing care.

d. analysis of quality data to identify opportunities for improving psychiatric-mental health nursing care.

e. formulation of recommendations to improve psychiatric-mental health nursing practice or patient outcomes.

f. implementation of activities to enhance the quality of psychiatric-mental health nursing practice.

g. participation on interdisciplinary teams that evaluate clinical practice or mental health services.

h. development of policies and procedures to improve safe, quality psychiatric-mental health care.

2. The psychiatric-mental health nurse seeks feedback from the patient and significant others about quality and outcomes of the patient's care.

3. The psychiatric-mental health nurse uses the results of quality-of-care activities to initiate changes throughout the mental health care delivery system, as appropriate.

Standard II. Performance Appraisal

The psychiatric-mental health nurse evaluates one's own psychiatric-mental health nursing practice in relation to professional practice standards and relevant statutes and regulations.

Rationale

The psychiatric-mental health nurse is accountable to the public for providing competent clinical care and has inherent responsibility as a professional to evaluate the role and performance of psychiatric-mental health nursing practice according to standards established by the profession.

Measurement Criteria

1. The psychiatric-mental health nurse engages in performance appraisal of one's own clinical practice and role performance with peers or supervisors on a regular basis, identifying areas of strength as well as areas for professional/practice development.

2. The psychiatric-mental health nurse seeks constructive feedback regarding one's own practice and role performance from peers, professional colleagues, patients, and others.

3. The psychiatric-mental health nurse takes action to achieve goals identified during performance appraisal and peer review, resulting in changes in practice and role performance.

4. The psychiatric-mental health nurse participates in peer review activities when possible.

5. The nurse's practice reflects knowledge of current professional practice standards, laws, and regulations.

Standard III. Education

The psychiatric-mental health nurse acquires and maintains current knowledge in nursing practice.

Rationale

The rapid expansion of knowledge pertaining to basic and behavioral sciences, technology, information systems, and research requires a commitment to learning throughout the psychiatric-mental health nurse's professional career. Formal education, continuing education, independent learning activities, and experiential and other learning activities are some of the means the psychiatric-mental health nurse uses to enhance nursing expertise and advance the profession.

Measurement Criteria

1. The psychiatric-mental health nurse participates in professional development activities to improve clinical knowledge, enhance role performance, and increase knowledge of professional issues.

2. The psychiatric-mental health nurse seeks experiences and independent learning activities to maintain and develop clinical skills.

3. The psychiatric-mental health nurse seeks additional knowledge and skills appropriate to the practice setting by participating in educational programs and activities, conferences, workshops, and interdisciplinary professional meetings.

4. The psychiatric-mental health nurse documents one's own educational activities.

5. The APRN-PMH maintains a mechanism for ongoing clinical supervision of practice.

Standard IV. Collegiality

The psychiatric-mental health nurse interacts with and contributes to the professional development of peers, health care clinicians, and others, as colleagues.

Rationale

The psychiatric-mental health nurse is responsible for sharing knowledge, research, and clinical information with colleagues, through formal and informal teaching methods, to enhance professional growth.

Measurement Criteria

1. The psychiatric-mental health nurse uses opportunities in practice to exchange knowledge, skills, and clinical observations with colleagues and others.

2. The psychiatric-mental health nurse assists others in identifying teaching/learning needs related to clinical care, role performance, and professional development.

3. The psychiatric-mental health nurse provides peers with constructive feedback regarding their practices.

4. The psychiatric-mental health nurse contributes to an environment that is conducive to education of nursing students, other health care students, and others as appropriate.

5. The psychiatric-mental health nurse actively promotes interdisciplinary collaboration.

6. The nurse contributes to a supportive and healthy work environment.

Standard V. Ethics

The psychiatric-mental health nurse's assessments, actions, and recommendations on behalf of patients are determined and implemented in an ethical manner.

Rationale

The public's trust and its right to humane psychiatric-mental health care are upheld by professional nursing practice. Ethical Standards describe a code of behaviors to guide professional practice. People with psychiatric-mental health needs are a vulnerable population. The foundation of psychiatric-mental health nursing practice is the development of a therapeutic relationship with the patient. Boundaries need to be established to safeguard the patient's well-being.

Measurement Criteria

1. The psychiatric-mental health nurse's practice is guided by the ANA *Code for Nurses.*

2. The psychiatric-mental health nurse establishes appropriate boundaries and maintains a therapeutic and professional relationship with patients at all times.

3. The psychiatric-mental health nurse maintains patient confidentiality within ethical, legal, and regulatory parameters.

4. The psychiatric-mental health nurse functions as a patient advocate.

5. The psychiatric-mental health nurse monitors any personal biases and seeks consultation or supervision as needed in order to deliver care in a nonjudgmental and nondiscriminatory manner sensitive to patient diversity.

6. The psychiatric-mental health nurse seeks to prevent ethical problems, identifies ethical dilemmas that occur within the practice environment, and seeks available resources to help resolve ethical dilemmas.

7. The psychiatric-mental health nurse reports abuse of patients' rights, and incompetent, unethical, and illegal practices.

8. The psychiatric-mental health nurse participates in the informed consent process (including the right to refuse) for patients' procedures, tests, treatments, and research participation, as appropriate.

9. The psychiatric-mental health nurse carefully monitors and manages self-disclosure in a therapeutic manner.

10. The psychiatric-mental health nurse does not promote or engage in intimate, sexual, or business relationships with current or former patients, and recognizes that to engage in such a relationship is unusual and an exception.

11. The psychiatric-mental health nurse guards against the exploitation of information furnished by the patient.

12. The psychiatric-mental health nurse is aware of and avoids the dangers of using the power inherent in the therapeutic relationship to influence the patient in ways not related to the treatment goals.

Standard VI. Collaboration

The psychiatric-mental health nurse collaborates with the patient, significant others, and health care clinicians in providing care.

Rationale

Psychiatric-mental health nursing practice requires a coordinated, ongoing interaction between consumers and clinicians to deliver comprehensive services to the patient and the community. Through the collaborative process, different abilities of health care clinicians are used to identify problems, communicate, plan and implement interventions, and evaluate mental health services.

Measurement Criteria

1. The psychiatric-mental health nurse collaborates with the patient, significant others, and other health care clinicians in the formulation of overall goals, plans, and decisions related to patient care and the delivery of mental health services.

2. The psychiatric-mental health nurse consults with other health care clinicians on patient care, as appropriate.

3. The psychiatric-mental health nurse makes referrals, including provisions for continuity of care, as needed.

4. The psychiatric-mental health nurse collaborates with other disciplines in teaching, consultation, management, and research activities.

Standard VII. Research

The psychiatric-mental health nurse contributes to nursing and mental health through the use of research methods and findings.

Rationale

Nurses in psychiatric-mental health nursing are responsible for contributing to the further development of the field of mental health by participating in research. At the basic level of practice, the psychiatric-mental health nurse uses research findings to improve clinical care and identifies clinical problems for research study. At the advanced level, the psychiatric-mental heath nurse engages and/or collaborates with others in the research process to discover, examine, and test knowledge, theories, and creative approaches to practice.

Measurement Criteria

1. The psychiatric-mental health nurse uses the best available evidence, preferably health-related research data, to develop the plan of care, interventions, and expected outcomes.

2. The psychiatric-mental health nurse participates in research activities as appropriate given the nurse's education, position, and practice environment. Such activities may include

    a. identifying clinical problems suitable for psychiatric-mental health nursing research.

    b. participating in data collection.

    c. participating on a unit, organization, or community research committee or program.

    d. sharing research findings with others through discussion groups, professional presentations, and publications

    e. conducting research as an individual investigator or as a member of a research team according to education and experience.

    f. critiquing research for applications to clinical practice.

    g. using research findings in the development of policies, procedures, and practice guidelines for patient care.

    h. consulting with research colleagues and experts.

3. The psychiatric-mental health nurse participates in clinical trials and human-subject protection activities as appropriate, recognizing the needs of the vulnerable subjects in the research study.

Standard VIII. Resource Utilization

The psychiatric-mental health nurse considers factors related to safety, effectiveness, and cost in planning and delivering patient care.

Rationale

The patient is entitled to psychiatric-mental health care that is safe, effective, and affordable. As the cost of health care increases, treatment decisions must be made in such a way as to maximize resources and maintain quality of care. The psychiatric-mental health nurse seeks to provide cost-effective, quality care by using the most appropriate resources and delegating care to the most appropriate, qualified health care clinician.

Measurement Criteria

1. The psychiatric-mental health nurse evaluates factors related to safety, effectiveness, availability, and cost when choosing between two or more practice options that result in the same expected patient outcome.

2. The psychiatric-mental health nurse assists the patient, family, or significant others in identifying and securing the appropriate and available services that address mental health needs.

3. The psychiatric-mental health nurse refers, assigns or delegates case activities as defined by the state practice act(s) and according to the knowledge and skills of the designated care giver.

4. If the psychiatric-mental health nurse refers, assigns, or delegates case activities, it is based on the mental health needs and conditions of the patient, the potential for harm, the stability of the patient's condition, the complexity of the task, and the predictability of the outcome.

5. The psychiatric-mental health nurse assists the patient, family, and/or significant others in becoming informed consumers about the benefits, risks, and costs of mental health treatment and care.

6. The psychiatric-mental health nurse documents the effects of resource utilization and changing patterns of mental health care delivery on psychiatric-mental health nursing and patient outcomes.

GLOSSARY

Activities of daily living—Self-care activities, such as eating, personal hygiene, dressing, recreational activities, and socialization, that are performed daily by healthy individuals as part of independent living. During periods of illness, individuals may not be able to perform some or all of these self-care activities.

Advanced practice registered nurse in psychiatric-mental health (APRN–PMH)—A licensed registered nurse (RN), educationally prepared at least at the master's degree level in the specialty, whose graduate level preparation is distinguished by a depth of knowledge of theory and practice, validated experience in clinical practice, and competence in advanced clinical nursing skills. The APRN-PMH focuses clinical practice on persons with diagnosed psychiatric disorders or those at risk of mental health disorders, and applies knowledge, skills, and experience autonomously to complex psychiatric-mental health problems.

Assessment—The systematic process of collecting relevant patient data for the purpose of determining actual or potential health problems and functional status. Methods used to obtain data include interviews, observations, physical examinations, review of records, and collaboration with colleagues.

Brief therapy—Treatment that focuses on the resolution of a specific problem or behavior in a limited number of sessions.

Case management—An intervention in which health care is integrated, coordinated, and advocated for individuals, families, and groups who require services. The aim of case management is to decrease fragmentation and ensure access to appropriate, individualized, and cost-effective care. As a case manager, the nurse has the authority and accountability required to negotiate with multiple clinicians and obtain diverse services.

Certification—The formal process by which clinical competence is validated in an area of practice.

Clinical supervision—The process in which one mental health professional seeks assistance from another to discuss therapeutic issues or to identify or clarify a concern or problem and to consider alternatives for problem resolution.

Counseling—A specific, time-limited interaction of a nurse with a patient, family, or group experiencing immediate or ongoing difficulties related to their health or well-being. The difficulty is investigated using a problem-solving approach for the purpose of understanding the experience and integrating it with other life experiences.

Crisis intervention—A short-term therapeutic process that focuses on the rapid resolution of an immediate crisis or emergency using available personnel, family, and/or environmental resources.

Diagnostic and Statistical Manual of Mental Disorders–IV Edition—Published by the American Psychiatric Association, the manual provides a listing of official diagnostic classifications for mental disorders. Each disorder is classified on one of five Axes—I and II include all clinical syndromes and personality disorders, III contains physical disorders, and IV and V provide information about psychosocial stressors and adaptive functioning.

Evidence-based—The collection, interpretation, and integration of valid, important, and applicable patient-reported, clinician-observed, and research-derived evidence. The best available evidence, moderated by patient circumstances and preferences, is applied to improve the quality of clinical judgments (McKibbon et al. 1996).

Family—Family of origin or significant others as identified by the patient.

Family and marital therapy—Approaches used to enhance the family's or couple's relationship and patterns of communication. Diagnoses, interventions, and outcomes emphasize the observable, interrelated behaviors that characterize the family or couple system.

Functional status—Level of the patient's ability to independently perform activities related to self-care, social relations, occupational functioning, and use of leisure time.

Holistic treatment—Provision of comprehensive care that identifies physical, emotional, social, economic, and spiritual needs as they relate to the individual's response to illness and to the ability to perform activities of daily living.

Illness trajectory—The course of the illness or chronic condition, which depends on the individual, the interventions utilized, and unpredictable events that occur during the illness' course.

Interventions—Nursing activities that promote and foster health, assess dysfunction, assist patients to regain or improve their coping abilities, and prevent further disabilities.

Managed care—Spans a broad continuum of entities, from the simple requirements of prior authorization for a service in an indemnity health insurance plan, to the assumption of all legal, financial, and organizational risks for the provision of a set of comprehensive benefits to a defined population. Also, the management of health care clinical services supplied by groups of providers with the aims of cost-effectiveness, quality, and accessibility.

Mental disorder/illness—A disturbance in thoughts or mood that causes maladaptive behavior, inability to cope with normal stresses, and/or impaired functioning. Etiology may include genetic, physical, chemical, biological, psychological, or sociocultural factors. Mental illness covers all mental disorders.

Mental functions—Characterized by alteration of thinking, mood, or behavior, or a combination of those.

Mental health—State of well-being in which individuals function well in society and are generally satisfied with their lives. State of successful performance of mental functions, resulting in productive activity, fulfilling relationships with other people, and the ability to adapt to change and to cope with adversity.

Mental health problems—Signs and symptoms of mental disorders with insufficient intensity or duration to meet criteria for any mental disorders.

Milieu therapy/therapeutic environment—A type of psychotherapy using the total environment to provide a therapeutic community. The emphasis is on developing the therapeutic potential of the setting by developing the physical surroundings, structured activities, a stable social structure, and cultural setting to promote interactions and personal growth.

Nurse practice act—State statute that defines the legal limits of practice for registered nurses.

Nursing practice standards—Authoritative statements that describe a level of care or performance, common to the profession of nursing, by which the quality of nursing can be judged. They include activities related to assessment, diagnosis, outcomes identification, planning, implementation, evaluation, quality of care, performance appraisal, education, collegiality, ethics, collaboration, research, and resource utilization.

Nursing process—A systematic and interactive problem-solving approach that includes individualized patient assessment, planning, implementation/intervention, and evaluation.

Outcomes—The patient's goal, or the result of interventions, that includes the degree of wellness and the continued need for care, medication, support, counseling, education.

Pathophysiology—The body's biological and physical processes that result in observable signs and symptoms.

Patient/patient system—The individual, family, group, or community for whom the nurse is providing formally specified services.

Phenomena of concern—Actual or potential mental problems that are of concern to psychiatric-mental health nurses.

Prescriptive authority—The statutory/regulatory authority to prescribe drugs and devices as a component of a profession's scope of practice.

Primary mental health care—A mode of service delivery that is initiated at the first point of contact with the mental health care system.

It involves the continuous and comprehensive mental health services necessary for promotion of optimal mental health, prevention of mental illness, intervention, health maintenance, and rehabilitation.

Professional code of ethics—Statement of ethical guidelines for nursing behavior that serves as a framework for decision making.

Psychiatric-mental health consultation—The process in which assistance is sought from a mental health professional about either the clinical care of a patient (client-centered consultation) or their own psychosocial or educational/skill development issues related to patient care issues (consultee-centered consultation), or the attainment of administrative expertise in either management of staff or program development (administrative consultation).

Psychiatric-mental health nursing—A specialized area of nursing practice that employs theories of human behavior as its science and the purposeful use of "self" as its art. It is the diagnosis and treatment of human responses to actual or potential mental disorders and their long-term effects. Interventions include the continuous and comprehensive primary mental health care services necessary for the promotion of optimal mental health, the prevention of mental illness, rehabilitation from mental disorders, and health maintenance.

Psychiatric-mental health registered nurse (RN-PMH)—A registered nurse who has a baccalaureate degree in nursing, has worked in the field of psychiatric-mental health nursing for a minimum of two years, and demonstrates competency in the skills of psychiatric-mental health nursing identified in this document.

Psychobiological interventions—Interventions (e.g., relaxation techniques, hypnosis, nutrition and dietary regulations, exercise, rest schedules, and psychopharmacological agents) used to improve well-being and functioning.

Psychopathology—The mind's biological and physical processes that result in observable signs and symptoms of mental disorder.

Psychopharmacological agents—Medications used to treat mental disorders.

Psychosocial domain—The range of diagnoses and treatments that are related to mental health, social status, and functional ability.

Psychotherapy—A formally structured, contractual relationship between the therapist and patient(s) for the purpose of effecting change in the patient system. Approaches include all generally accepted and respected methods of therapy, including individual therapy (play and other expressive therapies, insight therapy, behavioral therapy, cognitive therapy, and brief goal- or solution-oriented therapy), group therapy, couple/marital therapy, and family therapy.

Registered nurse (RN)—An individual educationally prepared in nursing and licensed by the state board of nursing to practice nursing in that state. Registered nurses may qualify for specialty practice at two levels—basic and advanced. These levels are differentiated by educational preparation, professional experience, type of practice, and certification.

Therapeutic community—The physical environment, patients, staff, and policies of the therapeutics facility, which have an influence on individuals functioning in the activities of daily living.

Therapeutic process—Use of the nurse-patient relationship and the nursing process to promote and maintain a patient's adaptive coping responses.

Therapeutic use of self—Individualized interventions in which the nurse uses theory and experiential knowledge along with self-awareness in assisting clients to explore their impact on others. The goal of therapeutic use of self is the facilitation of behavior change in the patient.

REFERENCES

1997 Behavioral managed care sourcebook: A comprehensive guide to mental health and substance abuse treatment delivery. 1996. New York: Faulkner & Gray.

Ahmed, S. M., and Maurana, C. A. 1999. Reaching out to the underserved: A collaborative partnership to provide health care. *Journal of the Health Care for the Poor and Underserved* 10:157–168.

American Nurses Association. 1999. *Competencies for telehealth technologies in nursing.* Washington, DC: American Nurses Association.

American Nurses Association. 1999. *Core principles on telehealth.* Washington, DC: American Nurses Association.

American Nurses Association. 1998. *Standards of clinical nursing practice.* 2nd ed. Washington, DC: American Nurses Association.

American Nurses Association. 1995. *Nursing's social policy statement.* Washington, DC: American Nurses Association.

American Nurses Association. 1994. *Statement on psychiatric-mental health clinical nursing practice and standards of psychiatric-mental health clinical nursing practice.* Washington, DC: American Nurses Association.

American Nurses Association. 1991. *Nursing's agenda for health care reform.* Kansas City, MO: American Nurses Association.

American Nurses Association. 1985. *Code for nurses with interpretive statements.* Kansas City, MO: American Nurses Association.

American Psychiatric Association. 1994. *Diagnostic and statistical manual of mental disorders–IV edition.* Washington, DC: American Psychiatric Association.

Boutain, D. M., and Olivares, S. A. 1999. Nurturing educational multiculturalism in psychosocial nursing: Creating new possibilities through inclusive conversations. *Journal of Psychosocial Nursing* 13:234–239.

Campbell, C. D., Musil, C. M., and Zauszniewski, J. A. 1998. Practice patterns of advanced practice psychiatric nurses. *Journal of the American Psychiatric Nurses Association* 4:111–120.

Caplan, G., and Caplan, R. B. 1993. *Mental health consultation and collaboration.* 1st ed. San Francisco: Jossey-Bass.

Carnevale, F. A. 1999. Toward a cultural conception of the self. *Journal of Psychosocial Nursing* 37:26–31.

Cohen, J. I. 2000. Stress and mental health: A biobehavioral perspective. *Issues in Mental Health Nursing* 21:185–202.

Collins, J. M. 1998. Caring for persons with developmental disabilities and psychiatric impairment. *Journal of the American Psychiatric Nurses Association* 4:90–102.

Dee, V., van Servellen, G., and Brecht, M-L. 1998. Managed behavioral health care patients and their nursing care problems, level of functioning, and impairment on discharge. *Journal of the American Psychiatric Nurses Association* 4:57–66.

Delaney, K. R., Chisholm, M., Clement, J., and Merwin, E. I. 1999. Trends in psychiatric mental health nursing education. *Archives of Psychiatric Nursing* 13:67–73.

Donaldson, S. K. 1997. The genetic social revolution and the professional status of nursing. *Nursing Outlook* 45:278–279.

Farnum, C. R., Zipple, A. M., Tyrrell, W., and Chittinanda, P. 1999. Health status & risk factors of people with severe and persistent mental illness. *Journal of Psychosocial Nursing* 37:16–21.

Flaskerud, J. H., and Wuerker, A. K. 1999. Mental health nursing in the 21st century. *Issues in Mental Health Nursing* 20:5–17.

Forchuck, C., Westwell, J., Martin, M-L., Bamber-Azzapardi, W., Kosterewa-Tolman, D., and Hux, M. 2000. The developing nurse-client relationship: Nurses' perspectives. *Journal of the American Psychiatric Nurses Association* 6:3–10.

Goldkuhle, U. 1999. Professional education for correctional nurses: A community-based partnership model. *Journal of Psychosocial Nursing* 37:38–44.

Haber, J. and Billings, C. V. 1995. Primary mental health care: A model for psychiatric-mental health nursing. *Journal of the American Psychiatric Nurses Association* 1:154–163.

Haber, J., and Billings, C. V. 1993. Primary mental health care: A vision for the future of psychiatric-mental health nursing. *ANA Council Perspectives* 2:154–163.

Kaas, M. J., and Markley, J. M. 1998. A national perspective on prescriptive authority for advanced practice psychiatric nurses. *Journal of the American Psychiatric Nurses Association* 4:190–198.

Kennedy, C. W., Polivka, B. J., and Chaudry, R. V. 1999. The role of public health nurses in service delivery to youth with mental disabilities. *Journal of the American Psychiatric Nurses Association* 5:177–184.

Krauss, J. 1993. *Health care reform: Essential mental health services.* Washington, DC: American Nurses Publishing.

Laffrey, S. C. and Kulbok, P. A. 1999. An integrative model for holistic community health nursing. *Journal of Holistic Nursing* 17:88–103.

Lindeke, L. L., and Chesney, M. L. 1999. Reimbursement realities of advanced practice nursing. *Nursing Outlook* 47:248–251.

McCabe, S., and Grover, S. 1999. Psychiatric nurse practitioners vs clinical nurse specialists: Moving from debate to action on the future of advanced practice nursing. *Archives of Psychiatric Nursing* 13:111–116.

McKibbon, K. A., Wilczynski, N., Hayward, R. S., Walker-Dilks, C. J., and Hayes, R. B. 1995. The medical literature as a resource for evidence based care. Working Paper from the Health Information Research Unit, McMaster University, Ontario, Canada.

Millholland, D. K. 1997. Telehealth: A tool for nursing practice. *Nursing Trends & Issues* 2:4.

Mohr, W. K. 1998. Managed care and mental health services: How we got to where we are. *Journal of the American Psychiatric Nurses Association* 4:153–161.

Mrazek, P. J. and Haggerty, R. J. 1994. *Reducing risks for mental disorders.* Washington, DC: National Academy Press.

Murray, C. J. L., and Lopez, A. D., eds. 1996. *The global burden of disease: A comprehensive assessment of mortality and disability from diseases, injuries, and risk factors in 1990 and projected to 2020.* Cambridge, MA: Harvard School of Public Health, on behalf of the World Health Organization and the World Bank.

North American Nursing Diagnosis Association. 1999. *Nursing diagnoses: Definitions and classification, 1999–2000.* Philadelphia: North American Nursing Diagnosis Association.

Palmer-Erbs, V. K. and Anthony, W. A. 1995. Incorporating psychiatric rehabilitation principles into psychiatric-mental health nursing practice: An opportunity to develop a full partnership among nurses, consumers, and families. *Journal of Psychosocial Nursing and Mental Health Services* 33:36–44.

Pascreta, J. V., Minarik, P. A., Caltaldo, J., Muller, B., and Scahill, L. 1999. Role diversification in the education of advanced practice psychiatric nurses. *Archives of Psychiatric Nursing* 13:48–60.

Pelletier, L. R., and Beaudin, C. L. 1999. Mental health services delivery and managed care. In *Advanced practice nursing in psychiatric and mental health care,* edited by C. A. Shea, R. L. Pelletier, E. C. Poster, G. W. Stuart, and M. P. Verhey. St. Louis: Mosby, pp. 37–72.

Pelletier, L. R., Poster, E. C., Shea, C. A., Stuart, G. W., and Verhey, M. P. 1999. Envisioning the future in mental health care. In *Advanced practice nursing in psychiatric and mental health care,* edited by C. A. Shea, R. L. Pelletier, E. C. Poster, G. W. Stuart, and M. P. Verhey. St. Louis: Mosby, pp. 547–562.

Pratt, J. R. 1999. Managing a culturally diverse work force. *Home Health Care Management & Practice* 11:67–69.

Rosedale, M. 1999. Managed care opens unlikely doors: Innovations in behavioral home health care. *Home Health Care Management & Practice* 11:45–48.

Sellin, S. C. 1999. Ethics and psychiatric home care. *Home Health Care Management & Practice* 11:1–7.

Shea, C. A. 1999. Careers in advanced practice psychiatric nursing. In *Advanced practice nursing in psychiatric and mental health care,* edited by C. A. Shea, R. L. Pelletier, E. C. Poster, G. W. Stuart, and M. P. Verhey. St. Louis: Mosby, pp. 1–34.

Shea, C. A., Pelletier, L. R., Poster, E. C., Stuart, G. W., and Verhey, M. P., eds. 1999. *Advanced practice nursing in psychiatric and mental health care.* St. Louis: Mosby.

Smith, G. B. 1999. Practice guidelines and outcome evaluation. In *Advanced practice nursing in psychiatric and mental health care,* edited by C. A. Shea, R. L. Pelletier, E. C. Poster, G. W. Stuart, and M. P. Verhey. St. Louis: Mosby, pp. 271–296.

Society for Education and Research in psychiatric-mental Health Nursing (SERPN). 1996. *Educational preparation for psychiatric-mental health nursing practice.* Pensacola, FL: SERPN.

Stuart, G. W. 1997. Recent changes and current issues in psychiatric nursing. In *Current issues in nursing.* 5th ed. Edited by J. C. McCloskey and H. K. Grace. St. Louis: Mosby.

Thomas, M. D., Brandt, P. A., and O'Connor, F. W. 1999. Preparing psychosocial nurse practitioners for health care delivery. *Archives of Psychiatric Nursing* 13:227–233.

U.S. Department of Health and Human Services, U.S. Public Health Service. 1998. *Healthy People 2010. National health promotion and disease prevention.* Washington, DC: U.S. Government Printing Office.

U.S. Department of Health and Human Services, U.S. Public Health Service. 1999. *Mental health: A report of the surgeon general.* Washington, DC: U.S. Government Printing Office.

Understanding Our Genetic Inheritance: The U.S. Human Genome Project, The First Five Years: Fiscal Years 1991–1995. 1990. DOE/ER-0452P, NIH Publication No. 90-1590.

Valentine, N. M. 1999. White House conference on mental health: Working for a healthier America. *Journal of the American Psychiatric Nurses Association* 5:167–171.

Verhey, M. P. 1999. Technology, information, and data management. In *Advanced practice nursing in psychiatric and mental health care,* edited by C. A. Shea, R. L. Pelletier, E. C. Poster, G. W. Stuart, and M. P. Verhey. St. Louis: Mosby, pp. 73–94.

Wallace, D. C., McGuire, S. L., Lee, H. T., and Sauter, M. 1999. Older Americans Act: Implications for nursing. *Nursing Outlook* 47:181–185.

Williams, C. A., Pesut, D. J., Boyd, M., Russell, S. S., Morrow, J., and Head, K. 1998. Toward an integration of competencies for advanced practice mental health nursing. *Journal of the American Psychiatric Nurses Association* 4:48–56.

World Health Organization.1993. *International classification of diseases.* 9th ed. Geneva: World Health Organization.

Wurzbach, M. E. 1998. Managed care: Moral conflicts for primary health care nurses. *Nursing Outlook* 46:62–66.

Wysoker, A. 1999.Thoughts for the millennium: The rights of the mentally ill. *Journal of the American Psychiatric Nurses Association* 5:197–200.

INDEX

Pages in *Scope and Standards of Psychiatric-Mental Health Nursing Practice* (2000) are marked by brackets [ ].

A

Accountability, 12, [78, 96]
  evidence-based practice, 12, [83]
  privatization and, [80]
  professional practice evaluation and, [120]
  quality of practice and, 45
  standards, 2
  state practice acts, 1, 20, [77, 95]
Acute care, 24
Addiction. *See* Substance abuse
Administration, 1, 4, [124]
Advanced practice psychiatric-mental health nursing, 3–5, 15, 19–20, [93–98]
  assessment, 29–30, [104–106]
  case management, [113]
  collaboration, 50, [123–124]
  collegiality, 49, [121–122]
  consultation, 43, [116]
  coordination of care, 36
  counseling, [110]
  defined, 19, 68, [127]
  diagnosis, 31, [106–107]
  education, 47, [120–121]
  ethics, 51, [122–123]
  evaluation, 44, [116–117]
  health teaching and health promotion, 37–38, [112–114 passim]
  implementation, 35, [109–110]
  leadership, 54–55
  milieu therapy, 39, [110–111]
  outcomes identification, 32, [107–108]
  pharmacological, biological, and integrative therapies, 40, [112]
  planning, 33–34, [108–109]
  prescriptive authority and treatment, 41, [115–116]
  professional practice evaluation, 48, [119–120]
  promotion of self-care, [111–112]
  psychotherapy, 42, [114–115]
  quality of practice, 45–46, [118–119]
  research, 52, [124–125]
  resource utilization, 53, [125–126]
  roles, 19–23, [94–98]
  See also Generalist practice psychiatric-mental health nursing; Psychiatric-mental health nursing
Advanced Practice Registered Nurse (APRN), 5, [79]
Advocacy, 18, 20, [85, 96, 101–102]
  ethics and, 51, [102, 123]
  for consumers and families, [80, 82]
  health teaching and health promotion, 37
  leadership and, 54
  psychopharmacology and, [92]
  psychotherapy and, 42
Age-related issues, *vii*, 6–7, 10, 11, [101]
  implementation and, 35
  See also Cultural competence
American Academy of Nursing, *vii*
American Nurses Association (ANA), *vii*, 3, 19, [76, 79, 86]
  Code of Ethics for Nurses with Interpretive Statements, 23, 51, [122]
  Nursing: Scope and Standards of Practice, *vii*
  Nursing's Social Policy Statement, 13–14
American Nurses Credentialing Center (ANCC), 3, 16, 19
  See also Certification and credentialing
American Psychiatric Association, [87]
American Psychiatric Nurses Association, *vii*, *viii*, [76]

Analysis. See Critical thinking, analysis, and synthesis

Assertive community treatment (ACT), 9, 25

Assessment, 14, 17, 25, [89, 95]
  consultation and, 22
  defined, 65, [127]
  diagnosis and, 31, [106]
  evaluation and, 44, [117]
  in evolving nursing roles, 3, 4, 5
  forensic, 27
  health teaching and health promotion, [90]
  implementation and, [110]
  milieu therapy and, 39
  pharmacological, biological, and integrative therapies, 40
  planning and, 33, 34, [87]
  prescriptive authority and treatment, 41
  screening and, [90]
  standard of practice, 29–30, [104–106]
  step in nursing process, 16, [88]
  See also Screening

Association of Child and Adolescent Psychiatric Nurses, [76]

B

Bailey, Harriet, 2

Balanced Budget Act, [81]

Barriers to mental health care, 8

Behavior, 2, 22, [87]
  at risk, 11, 15, 17, 38
  counseling and, [110]
  genetics and, 12–13
  planning and, 34

Body of knowledge, 2, [85]
  case management and, 21, [98]
  consultation and, 22
  education and, 5, 47, [96, 120, 121]
  evidence-based practice and, 13
  expansion of, [82–83, 94]
  health teaching and health promotion, 37, 38, [113]
  implementation and, 35
  levels of practice and, 16, 19–20, [93]
  milieu therapy and, [111]

outcomes identification and, [108]
  pharmacological, biological, and integrative therapies, 40, [91]
  planning and, 34
  psychotherapy and, 42, [115]
  quality of practice and, 45, [118]
  research and, [124]
  rural care and, 10

Brief therapy (defined), [127]
  See also Short-term care

Bureau of Health Professions, [79]

C

Caregiver (defined), 65

Care recipient. See Patient

Care standards. See Standards of practice

"Carve-in," [80]

"Carve-out," 7, [80]

Case management, 9–10, 11, [79]
  defined, [127]
  levels of practice, 18, 20, 21, [90–91, 96, 97]
  planning and, [109]
  standard of practice, [113]
  subspecialty practice, 23, [101]
  See also Coordination of care

Centers for Disease Control and Prevention (CDC), [79]

Certification and credentialing, [86, 93]
  defined, [127]
  education and, 3, 16, 19, [89]
  leadership and, 54
  quality of practice and, 46
  specialty practice and, 23

Client. See Patient

Clinical Nurse Specialist (CNS), 3–4, [79, 80]

Clinical settings. See Practice settings

Clinical supervision, 22–23
  defined, 65, [128]

Code of ethics (defined), 65

Code of Ethics for Nurses with Interpretive Statements, 23, 51, [122]
  See also Ethics

Collaboration, 9, 19, [82, 93–94, 96]
  collegiality and, [122]
  implementation and, 35
  milieu therapy and, 39, [110]

planning and, 33, [109]

research and, [124]

standard of professional performance, 50, [123–124]

violence and, [85]

See also Healthcare providers; Inter-disciplinary health care

Collegiality

diagnosis and, 31

ethics and, 51

implementation and, 35

professional practice evaluation and, 48, [120]

standard of professional performance, 49, [121–122]

Communication, 14, [83, 88]

advocacy and, [102]

assessment and, [104, 105]

collaboration and, 50, [124]

collegiality and, 49, [121]

consultation and, 43, [116]

counseling and, [110]

evaluation and, 44

leadership and, 55

milieu therapy and, [111]

pharmacological, biological, and integrative therapies, 40, [112]

psychotherapy and, 42

research and, 52, [125]

resource utilization and,

Community-based programs, 25, [82, 98–99]

advocacy and, [102]

assessment and, [104, 105]

coordination of care and, 36

crisis intervention and, 24

funding concerns, [81]

health teaching and health promotion, 25, 37, [92, 114]

implementation and, 35, [109]

levels of practice and, 19, 20, 21, [96, 97]

milieu therapy, [91]

origins, 3

in President's New Freedom Commission plan, 9

primary care and, [78]

research and, [125]

resource utilization and, 53

specialty practice, 23, [101]

Community Mental Health Centers Act, 3

Co-morbidity, 6, 10

defined, 65

diagnosis and, [106]

Competence assessment. *See* Certification and credentialing

Complementary therapies, 18, [82, 83, 91, 92]

in advance practice, [96]

assessment and, [105]

pharmacological, biological, and integrative therapies, 40, [112]

prescriptive authority and treatment, 41

Confidentiality, 21, 23, 27, [83, 97]

assessment and, 29, [105]

psychotherapy and, [114]

telehealth and, [100]

See also Ethics

Consultation, 4, 22, [83, 96, 97–98]

in advanced practice, 20

collaboration and, 50, [124]

defined, [131]

ethics and, 23

implementation and, [109]

primary care model, 26

research and, [125]

self-employment and, [100]

specialty practice, [101]

standard of practice, 43, [116]

telehealth and, 27, [100]

Continuity of care, 10, 14

case management and, [113]

collaboration and, 50, [124]

coordination of care and, 36

defined, 65

evaluation and, [117]

outcomes identification and, 32, [107]

planning and, 33, [109]

psychotherapy and, [115]

Coordination of care, [91]

implementation and, 35

leadership and, 54

standard of practice, 36

See also Interdisciplinary health care

Cost control, *vii*, 9, [77, 78, 79]
  community practice settings and, 24
  evaluation and, [117]
  outcomes identification and, 32, [107]
  planning and, 33, [109]
  prescriptive authority and
    treatment, 41
  quality of practice and, 46
  resource utilization and, 53, [125, 126]
Cost-effectiveness. *See* Cost control
Counseling, [93]
  defined, 65, [128]
  standard of practice, [110]
Credentialing. *See* Certification and
    credentialing
Crisis intervention, 24, [93]
  counseling and, [110]
  defined, 65, [128]
  implementation and, [109]
Criteria
  assessment, 29–30, [104–106]
  collaboration, 50, [123–124]
  collegiality, 49, [121–122]
  consultation, 43, [116]
  coordination of care, 36
  counseling, [110]
  defined, 65
  diagnosis, 31, [106–107]
  education, 47, [120–121]
  ethics, 51, [122–123]
  evaluation, 44, [116–117]
  health teaching and health promotion,
    37–38, [112–114 *passim*]
  implementation, 35, [109–110]
  leadership, 54–55
  milieu therapy, 39, [110–111]
  outcomes identification, 32, [107–108]
  pharmacological, biological, and
    integrative therapies, 40, [112]
  planning, 33–34, [108–109]
  prescriptive authority and
    treatment, 41, [115–116]
  professional practice evaluation, 48,
    [119–120]
  promotion of self-care, [111–112]
  psychotherapy, 42, [114–115]

  quality of practice, 45–46, [118–119]
  research, 52, [124–125]
  resource utilization, 53, [125–126]
Critical thinking, analysis, and
    synthesis, 9, 14, 19, [83]
  assessment and, 29, 30, [105, 106]
  case management, [91]
  consultation and, 43, [93, 116]
  coordination of care and, 36
  diagnosis and, 31
  evaluation and, 44, [117]
  health teaching and health
    promotion, 37, 38
  implementation and, [110]
  leadership and, 54
  planning and, 34, [109]
  professional practice evaluation and,
    48
  quality of practice and, 45, 46, [119]
  research and, 52
Cultural competence, 6, 21, [82, 84, 88]
  assessment and, 17, [104, 105]
  community-based care and, [97]
  consultation and, 22
  disparities in care, 7, 8
  ethics and, [102, 123]
  health teaching and health
    promotion, 37, 38, [92, 114]
  implementation and, 35
  levels of practice, 16, 18, [91, 92]
  milieu therapy and, 39, [111]
  outcomes identification and, 32
  planning and, 34
  promotion of self-care and, [111]
  screening and, [90]
  See also Age-related issues

D

Data collection, 17, [83, 90]
  assessment and, 29, [104]
  evaluation and, [116]
  quality of practice and, 45, [119]
  research and, 52, [125]
Data systems, 11–12
Decision-making, 11, 26, [82, 88, 102]
  collaboration and, 50, [124]

consultation and, 43, [116]
ethics and, [83, 103]
leadership and, 55
levels of practice and, 16, 20
professional practice evaluation and,
    48
screening and, [90]
Demographics of mental illness, 6–7,
    [83–85]
Diagnosis, 4, 14, 15, [83, 88, 95]
assessment and, 30, [105]
data system support, 11
defined, 65
evaluation and, 44, [117]
outcomes identification and, 32, [107]
planning and, 33
prescriptive authority and
    treatment, [115]
standard of practice, 31, [106–107]
step in nursing process, 16, [87]
Diagnostic and Statistical Manual of
    Mental Disorders, [87, 106, 128]
Disaster mental health, 28
Disparities in care, 6, 7–8, [80, 102]
Documentation, 27
assessment and, 30, [106]
collaboration and, 50
coordination of care and, 36
counseling and, [110]
diagnosis and, 31, [107]
education and, 47, [121]
evaluation and, 44, [117]
implementation and, 35, [110]
outcomes identification and, 32,
    [107, 108]
planning and, 33, [108, 109]
quality of practice and, 45
telehealth and, [100]

E

Economic issues. *See* Cost control
Education of psychiatric-mental health
    nurses, 2, 22, [78–79, 86]
collaboration and, 50, [124]
collegiality and, 49, [121, 122]
credentialing and, 3, 16, 19, [89]

graduate programs, 3, 4, 5
implementation and, [110]
leadership and, 12, 54
levels of practice, 1, 16, 19, 20, [77, 89,
    93, 96, 98]
lifelong learning, 12–13
quality of practice and, [119]
research and, 52, [125]
standard of professional
    performance, 47, [120–121]
subspecialty practice and, [101]
See also Mentoring; Professional
    development
Education of patients and families, 25,
    [79, 82, 85, 92]
case management, [91]
planning and, [108]
prescriptive authority and treatment,
    41
promotion of self-care and, [111]
telehealth and, [100]
See also Family; Health teaching and
    health promotion; Patient
End of life, 15, [88]
Environment (defined), 66
See also Practice environment
Environmental factors, 13
Ethics, 23, [82, 83, 102–103]
accountability and, 1
implementation and, [110]
leadership and, 54
psychotherapy and, 42
quality of practice and, 45
standard of professional
    performance, 51, [122–123]
See also Code of Ethics for Nurses
    with Interpretive Statements;
    Laws, statutes, and regulations
Evaluation, 14, 18, 23, [83, 88, 94]
assessment and, 30
collaboration and, [124]
defined, 66
health teaching and health promotion,
    [114]
implementation and, [109]
levels of practice, [90

Evaluation *(continued)*
     outcomes identification and, 32
     prescriptive authority and treatment,
          41
     psychotherapy and, 42
     quality of practice and, 46
     resource utilization and, 53
     standard of practice, 44, [116–117]
     step in nursing process, 16, [87]
Evidence-based practice, 6, 12–13, 14,
          [81, 83]
     assessment and, 29, 30
     consultation and, 43
     defined, 66, [128]
     education and, 47
     health teaching and health promotion,
          38, [113]
     implementation and, 35
     leadership and, 55
     nursing process and, 16
     outcomes identification and, 9, 32, [107]
     planning and, 34, [108]
     prescriptive authority and
          treatment, 41, [115]
     psychotherapy and, 42
     quality of practice and, 46
     telehealth, 27, [100]
     See also Research

F
Family
     assessment and, 29, 30, [104, 105]
     collaboration and, 50, [124]
     defined, 66, [128]
     diagnosis and, 31, [106, 107]
     evaluation and, 44, [117]
     milieu therapy and, 39
     outcomes identification and, 32
     planning and, 33, [108, 109]
     psychotherapy and, 42
     resource utilization and, 53, [126]
     See also Education of patients and
          families; Patient
Federation of Families, [82]
Financial issues. *See* Cost control
Forensic mental health, 27
Functional status (defined), [128]

G
Generalist practice psychiatric-mental
          health nursing, 16–19, [89–93]
     assessment, 29–30, [104–106]
     collaboration, 50, [123–124]
     collegiality, 49, [121–122]
     consultation, 43
     coordination of care, 36
     counseling, [110]
     diagnosis, 31, [106–107]
     education, 47, [120–121]
     ethics, 51, [122–123]
     evaluation, 44, [116–117]
     health teaching and health promotion,
          37–38, [112–114 *passim*]
     implementation, 35, [109–110]
     leadership, 54–55
     milieu therapy, 39, [110–111]
     outcomes identification, 32, [107–108]
     pharmacological, biological, and
          integrative therapies, 40, [112]
     planning, 33, [108–109]
     prescriptive authority and treatment,
          41
     professional practice evaluation, 48,
          [119–120]
     promotion of self-care, [111–112]
     quality of practice, 45–46, [118–119]
     research, 52, [124–125]
     resource utilization, 53, [125–126]
     roles, 18–19, [90–93]
     psychotherapy, 42
     See also Advanced practice
          psychiatric-mental health nursing;
          Psychiatric-mental health nursing
Genetics, 12, 19, [82–83]
Guidelines, [78, 83, 100]
     assessment and, 29
     defined, 66
     leadership and, 55
     outcomes identification and, 32
     professional practice evaluation and, 48
     quality of practice and, 45
     research and, [125]
     See also Standards of practice;
          Standards of professional
          performance

H

Health (defined), 66
Health teaching and health promotion,
     14, 15, [78, 86]
   community-based care and, 25
   consultation and, 22, [97]
   levels of practice, 17, 18, 19, [89, 90,
     92, 93, 94]
   pharmacological, biological, and
     integrative therapies, 40
   planning and, 33, 34
   program development, 21
   promotion of self-care and, [111]
   standard of practice, 37–38, [112–
     114 *passim*]
Healthcare policy, 5–6, 12, [77, 82]
   advocacy and, [102]
   evaluation and, 44
   leadership and, 55
   quality of practice and, 45, [119]
   research and, 52, [125]
Healthcare providers, 19, 20, 22, [96]
   assessment and, 29, [105]
   case management and, [113]
   collaboration and, 50, [123, 124]
   consultation and, 43
   defined, 66
   diagnosis and, 31, [107]
   evaluation and, 44, [117]
   implementation and, 35
   milieu therapy and, 39, [110]
   outcomes identification and, 32
   pharmacological, biological, and
     integrative therapies, 40
   planning and, 33, [108]
   See also Collaboration;
     Interdisciplinary health care;
     Referral
Healthcare team. *See* Collaboration;
     Interdisciplinary health care
Holistic care, 15, 19–20, 21, [82, 87, 91,
     94]
   assessment and, 29
   defined, 66, [129]
Home care, 25, 27, [82, 95, 99, 100]
   implementation and, [109]
   See also Practice settings

Hospitalization, 2, 3, 26, [99, 101]
   acute care, 24
   consultation and, 22, [97]
   crisis intervention, 24
   partial, 24–25
   See also Practice settings
Human resources. *See* Professional
     development

I

Illness (defined), 66
Illness trajectory (defined), [129]
Implementation, 14, 18, [88, 92]
   collaboration and, [124]
   coordination of care and, 36
   defined, 66
   evaluation and, 44
   health teaching and health
     promotion, [114]
   leadership and, 54
   outcomes identification and, 32
   planning and, 33
   quality of practice and, 46, [119]
   standard of practice, 35, [109–110]
   step in nursing process, 16, [87]
Information, 66
   See also Data collection
Institute of Medicine (IOM), 9
Insurance, 8, [82]
   See also Reimbursement
Integrative programs, 26
Intensive outpatient care, 24–25
Interdisciplinary health care, 6, 18
   assessment and, [105]
   collegiality and, 49, [122]
   coordination of care and, 36
   defined, 66
   education and, [121]
   ethics and, 51
   evaluation and, [117]
   implementation and, [110]
   outcomes identification and, [107]
   planning and, [109]
   quality of practice and, 46, [119]
   resource utilization and, 53
   See also Collaboration; Healthcare
     providers

Intermediate-term care, 24, [99]
    See also Practice settings
International Classification of Diseases,
    [87, 106]
International Nursing Society on
    Addictions, *vii*
International Society of Psychiatric
    Consultation Liaison Nurses, [76]
International Society of Psychiatric-
    Mental Health Nurses, *vii, viii*, [76]
Internet, 11, 38, [83]
Interventions, 9, [83, 85, 87]
    assessment and, [104]
    case management and, [90–91]
    collaboration and, [124]
    complementary therapies and, [92]
    defined, 67, [129]
    early, 21, 25
    evaluation and, [117]
    health teaching and health promotion,
        [114]
    implementation and, [109, 110]
    levels of practice, 18, 19, 20, [89, 96]
    milieu therapy and, 39
    pharmacological, biological, and
        integrative therapies, 40, [91–92]
    planning and, 34, [108, 109]
    prevention and, 11, 14
    promotion of self-care and, [112]
    psychotherapy and, 42
    research and, [125]
    See also Crisis intervention
Interviewing, [87]
    assessment and, 29, [104]
    consultation and, [116]
    counseling and, [110]
    diagnosis and, 31

K
Knowledge (defined), 67
Knowledge base. *See* Body of knowledge

L
Laws, statutes, and regulations, 1, 5, 27,
    [77, 95]
    assessment and, 29
    case management and, [97]

ethics and, 51, [123]
evaluation and, 44
implementation and, [109]
planning and, 33
prescriptive authority and treatment,
    41, [115]
professional practice evaluation and,
    48, [119, 120]
psychotherapy and, 42
resource utilization and, [126]
telehealth and, [100]
    See also Ethics
Leadership, *vii*, 2, 10, 19
    advocacy and, [102]
    coordination of care and, 36
    standard of professional performance,
        54–55
    transforming mental health care, 8–
        11
Licensing. *See* Certification and
    credentialing
Long-term care, 20, 24, 26, [96, 99]
    diagnosis and, 31
    See also Practice settings

M
McLean Asylum, 2
Managed care, 7, [129]
Management of health problems, 5, 14,
    15, [86–87]
Measurement criteria. *See* Criteria
Media, 11
Medicaid, [81]
Medicare, [81]
Mental disorder/illness (defined), 67,
    [129]
Mental health
    defined, 67, [129]
    demographics, 6–7, [83–85]
    physical health and, 7
Mental Hygiene Movement, 2
Mentoring
    collegiality and, 49
    leadership and, 54
Milieu therapy, [90, 91]
    defined, [130]
    standard of practice, 39, [110–111]

Models of primary care, 25–26
Multidisciplinary healthcare (defined),
    67
    See also Interdisciplinary health
        care

N
National Alliance for the Mentally Ill, 9,
    [82]
National Council on Disabilities, 9
National Institute of Mental Health, 3, 4
National Mental Health Act, 2, 3
National Organization of Nurse
    Practitioner Faculty, *vii*, 5
North American Nursing Diagnosis
    Association (NANDA), [87, 106]
Nurse practice act (defined), [130]
Nurse practitioner, 5, [79, 80]
Nursing care standards. *See* Standards
    of care
Nursing process
    defined, 67, [130]
    quality of practice and, 45
    steps, 16, [87]
    See also Standards of Practice
Nursing standards (defined), [130]
    See also Standards of practice;
        Standards of professional
        performance

O
Outcomes, 2, 11, [78, 83, 87]
    case management and, 10, 21
    collaboration and, 50
    defined, 67, [130]
    diagnosis and, 31, [107]
    ethics and, 51
    evaluation and, 14, 44, [116, 117]
    implementation and, 35, [110]
    planning and, 33, [95, 108, 109]
    prescriptive authority and treatment,
        41
    psychotherapy and, 42, [96]
    quality of practice and, 45, [119]
    recovery, 9, 10
    research and, [125]

resource utilization and, 53, [126]
    See also Outcomes identification
Outcomes identification, [88]
    standard of practice, 32, [107–108]
    step in nursing process, 16, [87]
    See also Outcomes
Outpatient care, 8, 9, 10, 22, 24–25
    See also Practice settings

P
Parents. *See* Family
Patient
    assessment and, 29, [104, 106]
    case management and, [113]
    collaboration and, 50, [123, 124]
    consultation and, 43, [116]
    coordination of care and, 36
    defined, 67, [130]
    diagnosis and, 31, [106, 107]
    ethics and, 51, [122]
    evaluation and, 44, [116, 117]
    health teaching and health
        promotion, 37
    milieu therapy and, 39, [110]
    outcomes identification and, 32, [107]
    pharmacological, biological, and
        integrative therapies, 40, [112]
    planning and, 33, [108, 109]
    prescriptive authority and
        treatment, 41, [116]
    professional practice evaluation and,
        48, [120]
    psychotherapy and, 42, [114, 115]
    quality of practice and, [119]
    relationship with nurse, 12, 18, 42, 51,
        [85, 93, 103, 109]
    resource utilization and, 53, [126]
    rights, 51, [82, 102, 123]
    See also Education of patients and
        families; Family
Patient-centered care, 8, 9, 13, 14, 22
    levels of practice, 18, 19, [97]
Peer review (defined), 67
Peplau, Hildegard, 3
Pew Health Professions Commission,
    [79]

Pharmacological, biological, and integrative therapies, 13, 26, [91–92]
  defined, 67, [131]
  implementation and, [109]
  standard of practice, 40, [112]
  See also Prescriptive authority and treatment; Psychopharmacology
Planning, 14, [83, 88, 91]
  assessment and, [104]
  collaboration and, 50, [124]
  consultation and, 43
  coordination of care and, 36
  defined, 67
  diagnosis and, 31, [107]
  evaluation and, 44, [117]
  health teaching and health promotion, [114]
  implementation and, 35, [109, 110]
  milieu therapy and, 39
  outcomes identification and, 32, [95, 107]
  research and, [125]
  resource utilization and, 53
  standard of practice, 33–34, [108–109]
  step in nursing process, 16, [87]
Policy. *See* Healthcare policy
Practice environment
  collegiality and, 49
  coordination of care and, 36
  leadership and, 54
  milieu therapy and, 39, [110, 111]
  See also Practice settings
Practice roles. *See* Roles in psychiatric-mental health nursing practice
Practice settings, 4–5, 22, 23–24, 27, [98–101]
  continuum of care, 14–15, 18
  See also Community-based programs; Home care; Hospitalization; Intermediate-term care; Long-term care; Outpatient care; Practice environment; Primary care; Residential care; Rural care; Short-term care
Preceptors. *See* Mentoring

Prescriptive authority and treatment, 18, 20, 27, [79, 94]
  assessment and, [105]
  defined, [130]
  education and, 4, 5
  standard of practice, 41, [115–116]
  See also Pharmacological, biological, and integrative therapies; Psychopharmacology
President's New Freedom Commission, *vii*, 9, 10
Prevention, 6, 11, 14, 15, [78, 87]
  community-based care and, 25
  counseling and, [110]
  genetics and, 13
  health teaching and health promotion, [113]
  levels of practice, 17, 19, [89, 94]
  planning and, 33
  primary care and, [86]
Primary care, 4, 5, 7, [78, 86–87]
  community-based, [97, 98]
  defined, 15, [86, 130]
  levels of practice, 15, 20, [94–95]
  models, 25–26
  self-employment and, 27, [100]
  See also Practice settings
Privacy. *See* Confidentiality
Process. *See* Nursing process
Professional development, 13, 22
  collegiality and, [121, 122]
  education and, [121]
  professional practice evaluation and, 48, [120]
  quality of practice and, [118]
  See also Education; Leadership
Professional organizations, 54
  See also American Nurses Association; American Psychiatric Nurses Association; International Society of Psychiatric-Mental Health Nurses
Professional performance. *See* Standards of professional performance
Professional practice evaluation
  collegiality and, 49

health teaching and health
   promotion, 37
   standard of professional
      performance, 48, [119–120]
Program development, 21
Promotion of self-care
   standard of practice, [111–112]
Psychiatric disorder (defined), 67
Psychiatric-mental health nursing
   body of knowledge, 2, 5, 10, 13, 16,
      19–20, 21, 22, 34, 35, 37, 38, 40, 42,
      45, 47, [82–83, 85, 91, 93, 94, 96, 98,
      108, 111, 113, 115, 118, 120, 121,
      124]
   certification, 3, 16, 19, 23, 46, 54, [86,
      89, 93, 127]
   characteristics,
   cultural competence, 6, 7, 8, 16, 17,
      18, 21, 22, 32, 34, 35, 37, 38, 39, [82,
      84, 88, 90, 91, 92, 97, 102, 103, 104,
      105, 111, 114]
   defined, 1, 13–14, [86, 131]
   education, 1, 2, 3, 4, 5, 12–13, 16, 19,
      20, 22, 47, 49, 50, 52, 54, [77, 78–79,
      86, 89, 93, 96, 98, 101, 110, 119,
      120–121, 122, 124, 125]
   ethics, 1, 10, 23, 42, 45, 51, 54, [77, 82,
      83, 102–103, 110, 122–123]
   healthcare providers and, 19, 20, 22,
      29, 31, 32, 33, 35, 39, 40, 43, 44, 50,
      66, [96, 105, 107, 108, 110, 113, 117,
      123, 124]
   history, 2–4
   phenomena of concern, 15–16
   practice environment, 36, 39, 49, 54,
      [110, 111]
   roles, 18–23, [88–98]
   scope of practice, 1–29, [86–103]
   standards of practice, 29–44, [104–117]
   standards of professional
      performance, 45–55, [118–126]
   trends, 5–13, [77–85]
   See also Advanced practice
      psychiatric-mental health nursing;
      Generalist practice psychiatric-
      mental health nursing

Psychiatric-mental health registered
   nurse (defined), [131]
Psychopathology (defined), [131]
Psychopharmacology, 4, 15, 21, [81, 83,
   88]
   defined, [131]
   levels of practice, 19, [90, 95, 96]
   planning and, 34
   restrictions on, [81]
   See also Pharmacological, biological,
      and integrative therapies;
      Prescriptive authority and
      treatment
Psychotherapy, 20–21, [96–97]
   defined, 68, [132]
   standard of practice, 42, [114–115]

Q
Quality of life, [93]
   diagnosis and, 31
   outcomes identification and, [107]
   planning and, 34, [108]
   promotion of self-care and, [112]
   quality of practice and, [119]
Quality of practice, 6, 11–12, [78, 79]
   collegiality and, 49
   defined, 67
   standard of professional
      performance, 45–46, [118–119]
   resource utilization and, 53, [126]

R
Recipient of care. See Patient
Recovery, 9–10, 13, 15, 16, 68, [92, 93]
Referral, 5, 15
   advanced practice, 19, 20, [94, 95, 96]
   collaboration and, 50, [124]
   planning and, [109]
   prescriptive authority and
      treatment, 41
   psychotherapy and, 42, [115]
   resource utilization and, [126]
   screening and, 14, [90]
   See also Collaboration; Coordination
      of care
Registered Nurse (defined), [132]

Regulatory issues. *See* Laws, statutes, and regulations
Rehabilitation, 9, 14, 15, [95]
  consultation and, 22, [97]
  levels of practice, 18, [87, 90, 93]
  long-term care, 24, [99]
  residential care, 25
Reimbursement, 4, 8, [80, 81, 94]
  psychotherapy and, [114]
Research, 1, 4, [83, 85, 86, 87]
  advanced practice, 20
  case management and, [97]
  collaboration and, 50, [124]
  collegiality and, [121]
  diagnosis and, [107]
  education and, 47, [120]
  ethics and, [123]
  evaluation and, [117]
  evidence-based practice and, 12, 14
  health teaching and health
    promotion, 37, [114]
  implementation and, [110]
  pharmacological, biological, and
    integrative therapies, 40, [112]
  planning and, 33, 34, [108, 109]
  psychotherapy and, 42
  quality of practice and, 46, [118]
  standard of professional
    performance, 52, [124–125]
  See also Evidence-based practice
Residential care, 25
  See also Practice settings
Resource utilization
  case management and, [113]
  health teaching and health promotion,
    37
  milieu therapy and, [111]
  standard of professional performance,
    53, [125–126]
Restraint, 23, [111]
Risk assessment, 13, 15, 21, [79, 85]
  case management, [91]
  diagnosis and, 31, [107]
  ethics and, 51
  health teaching and health promotion,
    38

implementation and, 35
leadership and, 54
outcomes identification and, 32
resource utilization and, 53, [126]
Robert Wood Johnson Foundation, [79]
Roles in psychiatric-mental health
    nursing practice, 18–23, [88–98]
  See also Advanced practice
    psychiatric-mental health nursing;
    Advanced Practice Registered
    Nurse; Clinical Nurse Specialist;
    Generalist practice psychiatric-
    mental health nursing; Psychiatric-
    mental health nursing; Registered
    Nurse
Rural care, 10
  See also Practice settings

S
Safety assurance, *vii*, 6, 13, 18, 23
  implementation and, 35, [110]
  milieu therapy and, 39, [111]
  planning and, 33
  quality of practice and, 46, [118, 119]
  resource utilization and, 53, [125,
    126]
Scientific findings. *See* Evidence-based
    practice; Research
*Scope and Standards of Psychiatric-
    Mental Health Nursing Practice*
    (2001), *vii*, [69–138]
Scope of practice, 1–29, [86–103]
Screening, 14, 18, 21, [90, 94, 95]
  implementation and, [109]
  See also Assessment
Self care and self-management, 15, 23,
    [87, 88, 90]
  health teaching and health
    promotion, 18, 37, [91]
  implementation and, [109]
  pharmacological, biological, and
    integrative therapies, 40
  planning and, [108]
  rehabilitation and, 93
  rural care, 10
Self-employment, 27, [100]

Settings. *See* Practice environment
Short-term care, 24, [81, 93]
    defined, [127]
    See also Practice settings
Significant others. *See* Family
Society for Education and Research in
        Psychiatric-Mental Health Nursing,
        [76]
Specialized areas of practice, 23–28
Specialty certification. *See* Certification
        and credentialing
Standard (defined), 67
Standards of care, *vii–viii*
    See also Standards of practice
Standards of practice, 29–44, [104–117]
    assessment, 29–30, [104–106]
    consultation, 43, [116]
    coordination of care, 36
    counseling, [110]
    diagnosis, 31, [106–107]
    evaluation, 44, [116–117]
    health teaching and health
        promotion, 37–38, [112–114
        passim]
    implementation, 35, [109–110]
    milieu therapy, 39, [110–111]
    outcomes identification, 32, [107–108]
    pharmacological, biological, and
        integrative therapies, 40, [112]
    planning, 33–34, [108–109]
    prescriptive authority and
        treatment, 41, [115–116]
    promotion of self-care, [111–112]
    psychotherapy, 42, [114–115]
Standards of professional performance,
        45–55, [118–126]
    collaboration, 50, [123–124]
    collegiality, 49, [121–122]
    education, 47, [120–121]
    ethics, 51, [122–123]
    leadership, 54–55
    professional practice evaluation, 48,
        [119–120]
    quality of practice, 45–46, [118–119]
    research, 52, [124–125]
    resource utilization, 53, [125–126]
Stigma, 8, [85, 102]
Subspecialty practice, [101]
Substance abuse, 4, 17, 18, 26, [81, 84,
        99, 101]
Substance Abuse and Mental Health
        Services Administration, 9
Supervisory activities, [98]
Synthesis. *See* Critical thinking, analysis,
        and synthesis

T
Taylor, Euphemia Jane, 2
Teaching. *See* Education; Health
        teaching and health promotion
Teams and teamwork. *See* Inter-
        disciplinary health care
Telehealth, 26–27, [78, 83, 100]
    implementation and, [109]
Terminology, 65–67
Therapeutic use of self, [89]
    defined, 68, [132]
Trends in psychiatric-mental health
        nursing practice, 5–13, [77–85]

U
Underserved populations, 10, [78]

W
W.K. Kellogg Foundation, [79]
Wald, Lillian, 2
Work environment. *See* Practice
        environment
World Health Organization (WHO), 6,
        [84]